panorama community
hospital
14850 roscoe boulevard
panorama city, california 91402

FUNDAMENTALS OF A PHERESIS PROGRAM

A Technical Workshop

Presented by the

Committee on Pheresis

AMERICAN ASSOCIATION OF BLOOD BANKS

Mention of specific commercial products or equipment by contributors to this American Association of Blood Banks symposium does not represent an endorsement of such products by the American Association of Blood Banks, nor does it necessarily indicate a preference for those products over other similar competitive products.

Efforts are made to have publications of the AABB consistent in regard to acceptable practices. However, as new developments in the practice and technology of blood banking occur, the Committee on Standards recommends changes when indicated from available information. It is not possible to revise each publication at the time each change is adopted. Thus, it is essential that the most recent edition of the Standards for Blood Banks and Transfusion Services be used as the ultimate reference in regard to current acceptable practices.

American Association of Blood Banks
Central Office, Suite 608
1828 L Street, N.W.
Washington, D.C. 20036

Edited by Jacob Nusbacher, MD, and Eugene M. Berkman, MD
with editorial assistance by Lois J. James and Rosanne Sheehan
ISBN No. 0-914404-45-8
First Printing
Printed in the United States of America

COMMITTEE ON PHERESIS

Eugene M. Berkman, MD, *Co-chairman*

Jacob Nusbacher, MD, *Co-chairman*

Asa Barnes, MD

Bruce A. Friedman, MD

Dennis Goldfinger, MD

F. Carl Grumet, MD

Douglas W. Heustis, MD

Jeffrey McCullough, MD

PREFACE

The introduction of pheresis activity into blood banks has proceeded at an unparalleled rate. This new activity has been characterized by a great deal of experimentation with regard to organizational problems, procedural nuances, the mitigation of donor and recipient hazards, and methods of evaluating product and procedure efficacy. Newcomers to the field, and even those already working in pheresis units, are often at a loss to find general and specific guidance on these matters in one place. The purpose of this workshop is to collate information on the current status of pheresis for the collection of components for transfusion. It is hoped that this material will be used as a resource in the day-to-day planning, work, and evaluation in pheresis centers.

In a workshop of this sort, it is inevitable that not everything can be covered. We have tried to address those issues that are fundamental to the successful operation of a pheresis program, but probably have overlooked important matters. All of the participants in this workshop have a large, personal experience in pheresis, and all have tried to present the current state of the art. However, personal preferences of the participants will be obvious or implied, and this is unavoidable. The careful reader will also discern occasional disagreements, even among the participants in this workshop. This merely reflects the fact that pheresis is still an evolving field and final answers — if there are such things — are not yet in.

J. Nusbacher, MD
E. M. Berkman, MD

CONTENTS

SUSAN K. WRIGHT, RN, Hemapheresis Nurse Supervisor,
The Johns Hopkins Oncology Center, The Johns Hopkins Hospital, Baltimore, Maryland

MARGARET C. MCELLIGOTT, SBB(ASCP), Transfusion Coordinator, The Blood Center of Southeastern Wisconsin, Milwaukee, Wisconsin

ALFRED J. KATZ, MD, Director, American Red Cross Blood Services, Connecticut Region, Farmington, Connecticut; and Associate Professor of Medicine, University of Connecticut School of Medicine

JACOB NUSBACHER, MD, Director, American Red Cross Blood Services, Rochester Region, Rochester, New York; and Associate Professor of Medicine, The University of Rochester School of Medicine

JAMES MACPHERSON, MS, Director of Special Projects, American Red Cross Blood Services, Rochester Region, Rochester, New York

LETTY KOTWAS, BS, RN, Pheresis Supervisor, American Red Cross, Northeastern New York Regional Blood Services, Albany, New York

JEFFREY MCCULLOUGH, MD, Director, American Red Cross Blood Services, St. Paul Region, St. Paul Minnesota; and Professor of Laboratory Medicine and Pathology, University of Minnesota School of Medicine

EUGENE M. BERKMAN, MD, Director of the Blood Bank,
New England Medical Center Hospital; and Associate
Professor of Medicine, Tufts University School of Medi-
cine, Boston, Massachusetts

JEROME B. ORLIN, MD, Fellow, Blood Bank and Division of
Hematology, New England Medical Center Hospital,
Boston, Massachusetts

Chapter 1

THE ORGANIZATION OF A HOSPITAL-BASED HEMAPHERESIS CENTER

Susan K. Wright, RN

THE NEED FOR BLOOD components for treatment of severely thrombocytopenic and granulocytopenic patients has escalated in the last six years. In response to that need, hemapheresis units have been developed in hospital blood banks, regional blood centers and, as in the case of Johns Hopkins Hospital, in oncology centers. As more methods of treating neoplastic diseases are developed, the patient need for blood component transfusion will only increase.

In established blood centers where component processing already was being performed, pheresis equipment frequently was added to expand plateletpheresis potential, with leukapheresis added at some later time. In many clinical units pheresis technology was first introduced for therapeutic hemapheresis and for investigational work in leukapheresis and leukotransfusion. At this institution the initial work was primarily leukapheresis. However, as the clinical need for leukotransfusion and platelet transfusion increased, the need for pheresis services dramatically increased (Fig 1).

The introduction of HLA-matched platelet support in 1977, and the recent rapid expansion of applications for therapeutic plasma exchange have further augmented the need for hemapheresis technology.

At Hopkins, it was decided to centralize all pheresis service into one specialized unit to avoid duplication of equipment and effort, and to standardize procedures. The Johns Hopkins Hemapheresis Center, therefore, was established in 1978 as an autonomous arm of the Blood Bank located in the Oncology Center. The unit currently operates six Haemonetics Model 30 celltrifuges and is responsible for planning and performing all pheresis procedures. Laboratory testing, storage, and issuing are performed by accredited laboratories within the Johns Hopkins Hospital.

This chapter describes the organizational structure and operation of this hospital-based hemapheresis center.

Transfusion Planning

Communication with Clinical Units

Communication is the single most important part of a mechanized society. As pheresis units have developed, the two major communication problems have been education concerning the medical indications for, and limitations of, component therapy, and dealing with busy patient services with multiple rotating physicians.

In any teaching institution patients are cared for by a team of doctors

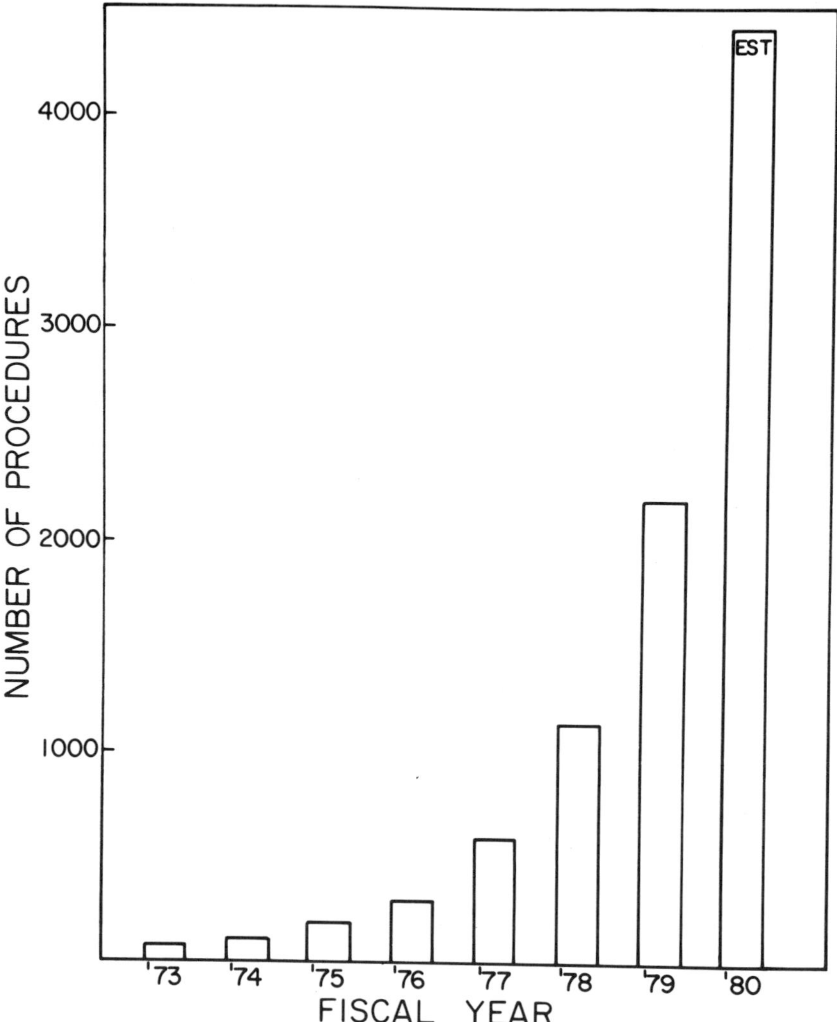

Fig 1. — Hemapheresis donation procedures fiscal 1973 through projected use fiscal 1980

including attending staff, fellows, residents, and interns. In the past, it has not been necessary for the medical staff to place a great deal of emphasis on transfusion planning because red cell transfusions were readily available. Consequently, this aspect of patient care traditionally has been given lower priority on a busy medical service. Because pheresis products have been limited by donor and machine availability and component shelf-life, good planning is necessary.

To achieve this, general guidelines for transfusion practices were established with the senior staff who admitted patients requiring pheresis services. To further refine planning, daily liaison was established with the attending physician and fellow. In this manner, lines of communication between the pheresis center and the clinical units are kept open.

Scheduling

One of the keys to efficient component transfusion has been to make maximum use of treatment protocols. Because cancer therapy, which results in severe aplasia, usually is given by protocol, it is possible to analyze the timing and degree of that aplasia in order to predict patient utilization of granulocytes and platelets. For example, the current protocol for adult acute nonlymphocytic leukemia in this institution is Day 1, 2, and 3, cytosine arabinoside by constant infusion, with daily doses of daunorubicin followed by cytosine arabinoside again on Days 8, 9 and 10. The resultant period of aplasia is between 28 and 35 days (Fig 2). Because of the severity of the aplasia, neutropenic patients usually are infected by Day 7 and proved nonresponsive to antibiotics by Day 14. Since the guidelines for granulocyte transfusion are refractory infections in severely neutropenic patients (<200 granulocytes/mm^3), it is possible to plan on granulocyte support from Day 14 through Day 28. Using these projections, a granulocyte transfusion schedule can be prepared for the majority of patients. By compiling each individual transfusion plan on a master sheet, a three-week schedule can be developed (Fig 3).

Likewise, thrombocytopenia, usually present on admission, can be expected to persist for the duration of the neutropenia. Maintaining a platelet count over 20,000/mm^3 usually requires transfusion of 3-5 units of platelets at least every two or three days. Therefore, a master schedule for random donor platelet transfusion also can be prepared.

All patients are HLA-typed prior to therapy, and any previously transfused patients are screened for lymphocytotoxic antibody against 15-20 random donors. Those patients who manifest either lymphocytotoxic antibody and/or poor platelet survival are monitored closely with one-hour posttransfusion platelet increments. When indicated, matched platelet support is scheduled and integrated into the pheresis schedule.

Using these standards for component support, it is possible to project platelet and granulocyte requirements. Every week, a three-week projection is made, and every Wednesday the plan is finalized for the following week. Patients are monitored daily for any change in condition which would necessitate changing their transfusion plan. In this manner the Hemapheresis Unit can plan to act on patient needs, rather than to react to unplanned blood orders.

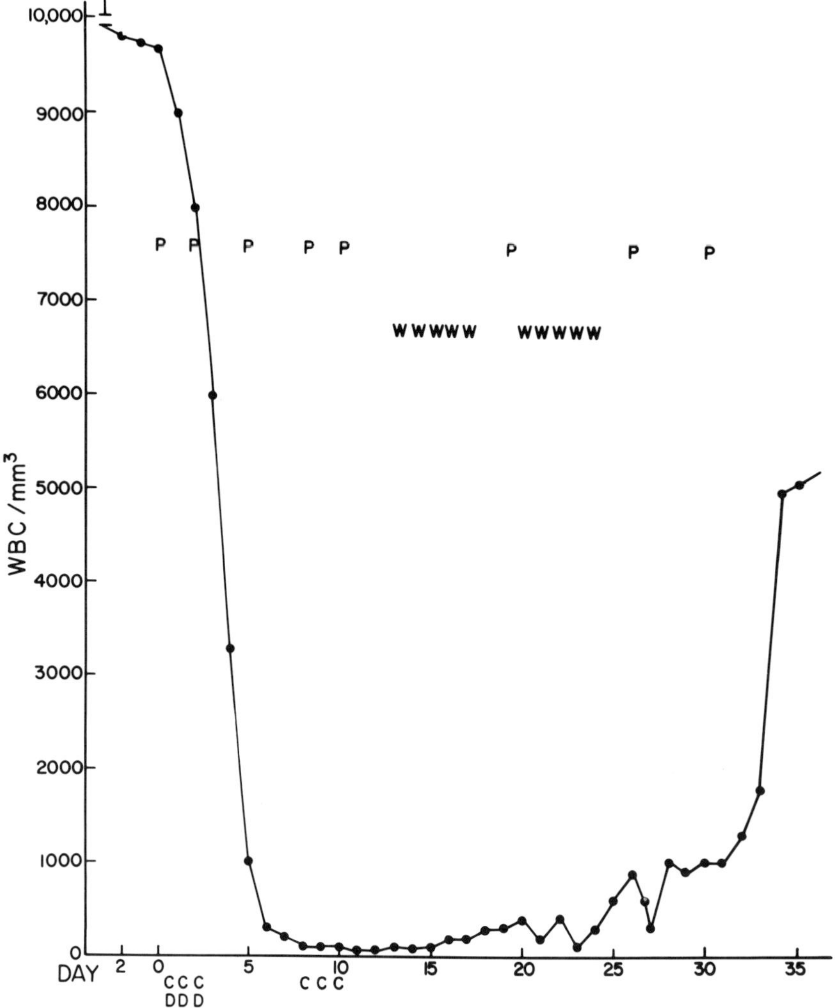

Fig 2. — Estimated component use in acute leukemia. C = Cytosine Arabinoside; D = Daunorubicin; W = White Cell Transfusion; P = Platelet Transfusion

The Component Transfusion Group consists of the pheresis supervisor, donor room leader, medical director, and two physician's assistants (Fig 4). All physicians direct their requests for blood components through the physician's assistants. Any nonstandard request is presented to the medical director.

The function of the Component Transfusion Group is fourfold:

1) To keep open lines of communication between the patient services and Hemapheresis by attending patient rounds,
2) To generate and document a data base about platelet transfusion efficacy,
3) To formulate utilization estimates based on previous transfusion statistics,
4) To allocate individual platelet transfusions according to previously established guidelines.

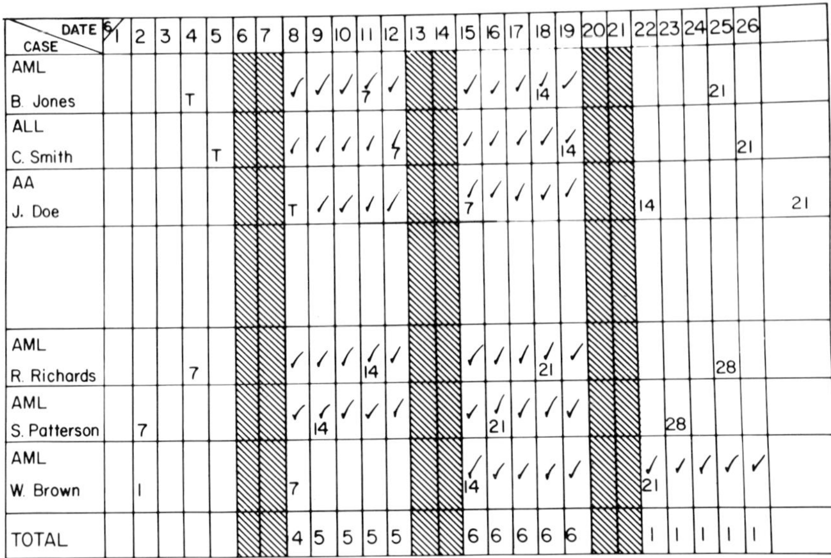

Fig 3. — Cumulative leukotransfusion planning sheet. T = transplant day, Number = day of protocol; √ = planned leukotransfusion

At a daily meeting held after patient rounds are finished and morning platelet counts are available, the most recent transfusion data on each patient are reviewed. Patient problems such as bleeding, fever, infection and in vitro evidence of alloimmunity are discussed and transfusion planning is modified to meet clinical requirements.

An interdisciplinary transfusion planning conference is held every Monday afternoon. The Component Transfusion Group meets with representatives from the Blood Bank, HLA Laboratory, and any physician who wants to discuss the component needs of his patients. The purpose of this meeting is to address patients with transfusion problems. This is a formal information-sharing session for setting policy and preparing patient transfusion plans. The end result of these meetings is better patient care and better understanding between services with a common goal.

Applicability

This type of transfusion planning requires a major commitment of staff time, compensated for by better patient care and more efficient func-

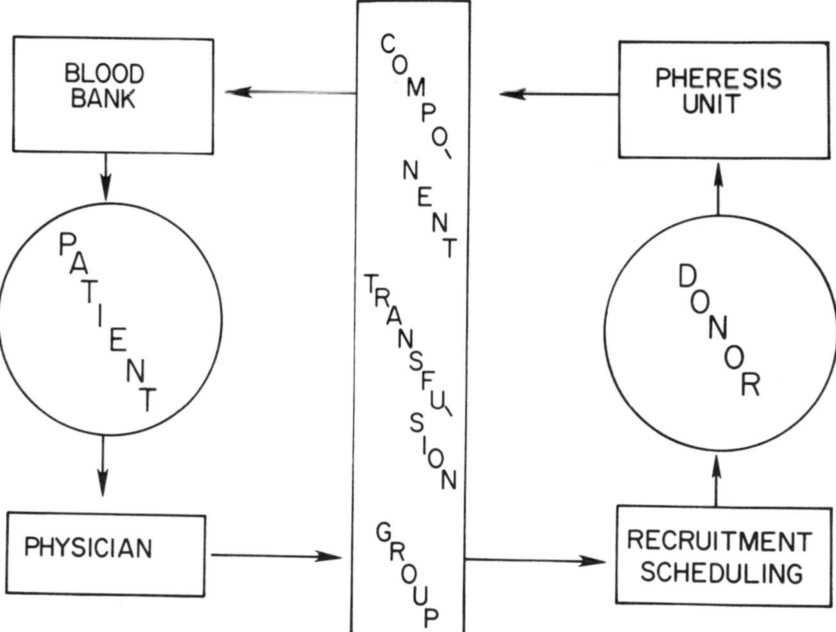

Fig 4. — Component Transfusion Services: transfusion, evaluation, planning and production

tioning of the pheresis unit. It is rare that granulocyte units are not transfused; platelet outdating is kept to less than 15% in an institution supporting 30 patients daily and transfusing 2,000 units of platelets per month.

While smaller patient services do not need such a large staff, the principles of efficient planning still should apply. Standards of transfusion practice should be established between the pheresis service and the primary care physicians using the service. Support strategies can be established after there is an understanding of the myelosuppressive dynamics of each treatment regimen or protocol. The pheresis unit should then be consulted as early as possible about any patient who may require support. Daily liaison can be initiated to establish the data base necessary to guide efficient transfusion support.

Donor Recruitment

Donor recruitment is a concern for any blood bank system. Pheresis units established in areas with existing whole blood donor programs have tapped their existing donor pools for candidates for pheresis. Good visibility in a donor room can, in itself, stimulate questions and donors from the whole blood donor program.

Those units which started in clinical areas generally have depended upon families to provide the necessary donors. The advantages of using family members are that they are highly motivated to donate, and it is often psychologically therapeutic for them to be able to do something to aid their loved one in a situation where they feel helpless. In addition, family members may be a close HLA-match.

At Hopkins, every leukemic and bone marrow transplant patient is interviewed upon admission to ascertain whether he/she will be able to provide donors. Patients who cannot supply donors are supported from a pool of 500 random donors.

As more expertise was gained in transfusing platelets, it became evident that a larger random donor pool was necessary in order to transfuse HLA-matched platelets to patients who are alloimmunized. Therefore, Hopkins is just getting into the area of large-scale donor recruitment using technics found successful at other institutions. Newspaper articles and public service announcements on radio and television have yielded many donors. However, work with the first departments of Baltimore City and the surrounding counties has yielded many more donors. Because of their personal altruism and odd work schedule, firefighters make excellent pheresis donors. However, it is necessary to remember that they are members of a hazardous profession.

Our approach to prospective donors is one of education. With the assistance of a slide/tape show, it is possible to address an audience about the need and the procedure, while at the same time stimulating them to become pheresis donors.

During donation, the machine operator reinforces the teaching the donor already has received, explaining the importance of the blood components being donated. If the donor is not a member of the random donor pool, he is encouraged to join. If a member, he is encouraged to bring a buddy to Pheresis; the "Buddy System" hasn't doubled the size of our donor pool, but it has augmented it.

There are many ways to reinforce and encourage donors: "Super Donor" tee shirts and pins, plaques and mugs for multiple donations, wall hangings in the donor room for multiple donors, to name just a few. Greeting cards for holidays and birthdays also are effective. To let donors know that their effort is appreciated, the Hopkins Hemapheresis Unit often uses a quote by Edwin Markham:

> "There is a destiny that makes us brothers —
>   None goes his way alone;
>   All that we send into the lives of others
>   Comes back into our own."

A donor advisory committee consisting of donors and staff has been used successfully in many blood banks and pheresis units. The purpose of the committee is to identify ways to stimulate more donors and to reinforce existing ones.

We feel that the process of recruiting pheresis donors should be a total community effort, organized to educate the public to the need and to provide donors for all programs. Pheresis donors should be recruited only from within the active red cell donor pool if the program is large enough to handle the loss. Otherwise they should be stimulated from a whole new group of people so that the total patient need can be met.

Physical Plan

A pheresis unit has many requirements for physical layout:
1. Easy accessibility for donors
2. Pleasant atmosphere
3. Quietude
4. Good visibility for easy supervision of personnel and donors
5. Private area for patient procedures
6. Adequate space for:
   a) confidential interviewing
   b) storage
   c) product sampling
   d) canteen

However, pheresis units frequently have been added to already crowded facilities, adapting needs to available space. The Hopkins hemapheresis donor room is 40×20 feet. Contained in that area are five beds and five Haemonetics Model 30s, a donor nourishment area, a blood processing area, and a small office area for the nurse supervisor.

The floor is covered with carpeting to reduce noise, the color television has ear phones, and the room is decorated with plants and wall hangings to create a pleasant, non-hospital-like atmosphere for donors. The open space allows for easy supervision of personnel and procedures.

Because this area is not large enough for a projected seven machines, and it affords no private area for patient procedures, there is another pheresis area 23×15 feet which contains two beds, space for two Model 30s and some office space.

The recruitment office is an area 20×18 feet divided into four cubicles. Three are for confidential donor interviewing; the fourth is a waiting area (where a secretary works).

Including office space, the Hemapheresis Center occupies 1,720 square feet of floor space. This is an average of 245 square feet per machine. In spite of the size, the area is cramped and, in some ways, inadequate. Probably 300 square feet per machine is a better estimate of necessary space. The type of pheresis equipment and donor chairs used, plus the availability of shared facilities, can modify the space requirement at other hospitals.

Staffing

The technical staff of pheresis units comes from varied educational backgrounds. Medical technologists, medical technicians, machine or pheresis technicians, and nurses are all performing pheresis. This seems to be dependent upon where the unit was started and whether its purpose was research or service.

We selected nurses as the mainstay of our staff because of their ability to deal with people and their background in observation skill, history-taking, sterile technic, fluid and electrolyte balance, and venous access. However, they have a definite lack of education in blood banking and donor criteria; these are addressed as part of the orientation program. We have to retrain many nurses to be perfectionists, a characteristic which is essential in blood banking. To supplement the staff, we have two on-the-job-trained machine technicians with a work background in patient care.

Leadership

The staff of the Hemapheresis Unit comes under the direct supervision of the nurse supervisor (Fig 5). Functional areas within the Pheresis Unit are assigned individual leaders. Our original staffing plan was to have a nurse leader for each area, and then to have those leaders rotate through different areas every three or four months. It was felt that the jobs were not of equal pressure, and rotation would allow time for personal research and development. Also, there was a concern that doing only one aspect of the job would be boring after a period of time. However, we discovered that our leaders have innate talents for doing different types of work and, while it is possible for them to function in other positions, they are much more productive in the area in which they are most comfortable. As long as they are growing within their jobs and not bored with routine, we will continue to function with leaders scheduled only in their area of expertise. However, if it becomes necessary for job stimulation at some later time, we will initiate leader rotation.

Donor Room

The donor room leader is a nurse experienced in all types of pheresis, donor recruitment, and scheduling. Her role includes teaching, assigning work, donor acceptance/rejection, donor monitoring, donor reaction

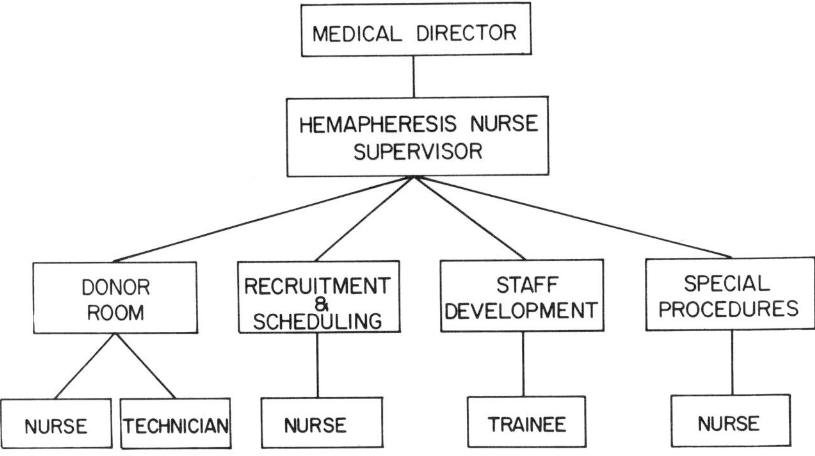

Fig 5. — Organizational diagram

management, maintenance of records, and assuring the smooth operation of the donor room.

Answering to her for their performance in the donor room are the technicians and nurses. Nurses within the donor room perform histories, evaluate vital signs, perform venipunctures, set up machines and run them for component collection, do blood processing and labeling, record keeping and charting. They are also cross-trained in donor recruitment, work-up, and scheduling. Machine technicians set up and run machines for component collection, do blood processing and labeling, and machine maintenance.

Everyone is responsible for the day-to-day tasks necessary for keeping the room going, such as cleaning, stocking, filing, special projects for testing new equipment, and improving procedures.

Donor Recruitment and Scheduling

The donor recruitment leader is experienced in pheresis. Her responsibility is to see that the proper donors are scheduled for the proper patient on the days when they will be needed.

She makes our initial contact with the patient and the family, explaining what we do and how we interact with the floor staff in the patient's care. She asks for assistance from family and friends in providing donors for the patient. She is responsible for the potential donor education concerning pheresis, informed consent, health history, and initial blood screening. After each chart is screened by the medical director, donors are called and scheduled for donation.

By Wednesday of each week, a decision is made about the patients who are to receive white cell transfusions the next week. Donors are scheduled according to HLA-matched platelet need, white cell need, projected single donor platelet usage, therapeutic procedures necessary, available staffing, and machine time.

A nurse from the pheresis staff rotates though the donor recruitment area for a two- or three-week stay, depending on the work load. All pheresis nurses are trained to work in this area. Since the recruitment leader is the person calling donors and scheduling them for donation, she makes a point of coming to the donor room at least twice a day. She personally thanks each donor for coming, thus reinforcing her telephone voice with personal contact.

Special Procedures

The "special procedures" leader is a nurse totally qualified to relieve the leader in either of the other areas. She is in charge of all patient procedures, making the initial contact with a patient, assessing venous access, and explaining the procedure in order to obtain an informed consent. She is responsible for the patient during pheresis and for follow-up afterwards. She is also responsible for special projects, such as bone marrow processing, and for developing new protocols for ways of adapting or improving procedures. Additional staff works with the "special procedures" leader as is necessary, depending upon scheduled procedures. All staff is trained to work in this area.

Staff Development

The "staff development" leader is responsible for training new staff by using a one-on-one teaching method, with our pheresis manual and self-learning packages as reinforcement. It takes three months of daily setting up the machine, running donors, processing blood, and doing the accompanying paperwork, before a trainee is a good, independent machine operator for component collection. At least the first three weeks require constant attention and reinforcement from an instructor. Once the machine operator is comfortable with the machine and its capabilities, plus the donor and possible donor reactions, it is easy to adapt the knowledge to other types of pheresis procedures.

After six months of education and experience, we consider a nurse completely trained: able to understand the disease processes for which we transfuse and pherese; able to identify, educate, evaluate and pherese donors; and able to manage either patients or donors during pheresis. Our staff development program also includes educational programs by our medical director, Blood Bank, and HLA Typing Lab.

Operations Staff

A pheresis nurse or technician is a very special person, combining the ability to interact well with people with being a teacher, a mechanic, and a perfectionist.

Staff Scheduling

Our unit, like similar units at most institutions, believes that a machine operator should be with a donor at all times during a donation procedure. Ostensibly, she/he is there to run the machine, but the operator's primary function is to observe the donor for untoward reactions, monitor the pheresis equipment for proper functioning, and make the donor comfortable during donation.

When a nurse is assigned a donor at Hopkins, she is responsible for all of the preparative paperwork, evaluation of the donor by history and vital signs, setting up the machine, and running the donor. After the run, she is responsible for processing and sampling the products, calculating the total cell yield, labeling the blood, and finishing the chart and the log for that donation.

Experience has shown that one operator can do one-and-one-half white cell runs, or two platelet runs, per day with the accompanying paperwork and blood processing. Therefore, the basis for maximum workload is one and one-half or two times the number of operators working in the donor room.

In therapeutic procedures, on the other hand, the patient is not as stable as a healthy donor, so the staffing is a machine operator plus a nurse to observe the patient and keep him/her in fluid balance. If, after many exchanges, the patient is comfortable with the procedure and it is documented that he is stable during pheresis, one experienced nurse can handle the procedure.

With this as a basis for staffing as it relates to workload, it is then possible to calculate the total number of machine operators which are necessary. Using the best estimates of the principal investigators for projected patient treatment, and statistics gathered in the past for length of stay and platelet and granulocyte utilization by diagnosis, it is possible to project the annual need for pheresis components. Projected utilization for fiscal 1980 is 1,680 leukaphereses, 15,000 units of single donor platelets, 2,000 units of HLA-matched platelets, and 600 therapeutic procedures. It is now necessary to consider the number of staff required for the projected therapeutic and research procedures, plus the number of supervisors and recruitment personnel necessary to keep up with the workload, in order to calculate the total projected size of our pheresis unit.

Staff Motivation

One part of staffing essential to address is motivation. A large amount of time is spent in thinking of ways to motivate donors and not enough consideration is given to staff motivation. In order to have a good pheresis unit, it is necessary to keep a staff for which time and effort in training already have been invested. Rotation through the recruitment area allows patient interaction that usually does not occur in the donor room. Case assignments for plasma exchange allow for involvement of staff in the progress of a patient. Continuing education programs, designed so that pheresis personnel can see how their role interacts with the patient and with research projects, are extremely important.

Physician Coverage

The medical director or a covering physician stays within the confines of the four floors of the Oncology Center during all pheresis procedures. He is available to administer emergency medical care or to evaluate any nonstandard donor reaction. He carries a radio beeper which is used only for pheresis emergencies. Instead of responding by telephone, he comes quickly to the Pheresis Unit.

Patient procedures require closer supervision. During the first hour of a patient's first procedure, the physician is in the room or immediate area. If, after that hour, the patient seems to be tolerating the procedure well, the physician is available for any problems via his beeper.

The standards of the American Association of Blood Blanks require that a physician be available within ten minutes for whole blood donation, and many pheresis centers operate on this criteria. However, we consider pheresis a more complex procedure with some poorly defined variables, which can lead to potentially serious adverse donor reactions, including arrythmias, hypovolemia, and mechanical malfunctions. The covering physician is considered the doctor for each donor. He is responsible for medical clearance for donation, treatment of any adverse reactions, and follow-up and review of all donor data. For these reasons it is necessary for him to be in the area.

Essential Support Systems

Data Processing

Contained within the computer of the Johns Hopkins Oncology Center is a system for pheresis. The profile on every donor includes pertinent information such as name, address, social security number, birthdate, ABO and HLA types, and a listing of all donations, including the type and quantity of cells retrieved.

After a donation, all of the pertinent information is fed into the computer; the date and type of donation is recorded on the donor's profile. The products appear on an inventory sheet together with the HLA type, ABO type, quantity of cells, and the results of the lymphocytotoxicity testing with patients who are having alloimmunity problems. As the products are transfused, they are automatically removed from the inventory and placed on the patient's transfusion record. With the added information of a one-hour postplatelet count, the computer then will calculate the platelet increment.

The computer has the ability to give us listings of the best matched donors according to HLA type by inserting the HLA type of the patient. Also, because of the types of data put into the computer about each run, we can retrieve data by machine operator, machine number, and donation day or donor, giving us the ability to compare cell yields by machine, operator, or date. In order to coordinate this system with our own, it is necessary for us to have, working within our system, a data coordinator familiar with, and able to integrate with, data processing.

Blood Bank

It is essential for a pheresis unit to have excellent communication and interaction with a blood bank. The Johns Hopkins Blood Bank does all red cell typing, crossmatching, RPR and RIA testing, storage, and issuing of our pheresis products. Because of the short storage time of pheresis products, it is necessary for them to be able to do rapid and accurate hepatitis and syphilis testing.

HLA Typing Lab

In order to transfuse white cells and platelets effectively, it is necessary to have the support of an HLA laboratory for typing and lymphocytoxic crossmatching. The expertise in patient transfusion and donor identification is essential.

Hematology and Chemistry Laboratories

Our Oncology Department finds it necessary to have a hematology laboratory on the premises. This is a distinct advantage because our laboratory work is done on the same floor as the donor room. The laboratory has to adapt to pheresis products by doing manual counts and wet prep differentials. Hematology and chemistry laboratory support is essential for donor, patient, and product management.

Clinical Engineering

To make a piece of machinery run smoothly day after day, it is essential to have some on-the-spot expertise in the mechanics of the hardware. With the new federal regulations for high technology medical equipment, expertise in clinical engineering is necessary. Monthly quality control checks on pumps, centrifuge, and solenoids help to maintain hardware.

Administration

Good fiscal policy is extremely important for the successful operation of a blood bank system. Because Hopkins is a private institution in a state with rate control, it was necessary to develop a management tool which could be used to monitor fiscal performance.

Ratios developed among the various products and procedures were based on their individual utilization of resources. Using 5.5×10^{10} as one equivalent unit of platelets, 8.5 equivalent units can be retrieved from one plateletpheresis. If one unit of platelets is considered to be the Pheresis Relative Value Unit, it then is possible to calculate the number of relative value units for any pheresis procedure by comparing the direct costs for each procedure (Table 1).

During leukapheresis, it is possible to retrieve six units of platelets separated from the white cells. These units of platelets can be transfused to another patient, decreasing the cost of the white cell transfusions.

The Pheresis Relative Value Unit has some easily identifiable benefits:

1. Budgeting and cost analysis are simplified.
2. Prices can be changed easily, maintaining the proper proportion among products.

3. Production can be monitored even though the ratio of platelet-pheresis to leukapheresis is different.
4. New services can be added without establishing a new charge system.

Forms

Documentation is an integral part of any blood bank system. A chart is created on each prospective donor at the time of initial work-up. After a detailed description of hemapheresis, the donor is asked to sign an informed consent form (Fig 6). A health history is taken, conforming to the standards of the American Association of Blood Banks, but also asking more in-depth questions in such areas as cardiac and renal history. The

Table 1. — Pheresis Relative Value Unit (RVU): Ratio of consumed resources

RESOURCES	PLATELETS	GRANULOCYTES
Surgical supplies	$ 72.32	$ 108.76
Laboratory testing (donor and product)	87.00	183.00
Nursing / Tech. staff	26.00	39.00
Difficulty factor	4.21	16.84
Total resource consumption	189.53	347.60
Units	8.5	1
Resource consumption per Unit	$ 22.30	$ 347.60
Ratio	1	15.6
Value of Platelets from Granulocyte run	–	(6.0)
Pheresis R.V.U.	1	9.6

history, informed consent, and laboratory test results are put into individual folders with a front sheet (Fig 7) which shows pertinent laboratory and run data. Once the donor is accepted by the recruitment nurse, the chart is reviewed by the medical director before donation. This donor chart is analogous to a patient's medical records and can be easily cross-referenced with the run data and daily log through the identifying unit number.

At the time of donation, another health history is taken in conformance to the standards of the American Association of Blood Banks and a release is signed for the use of the blood products. After donation, the daily history, release form, and the laboratory data go into the chart with the yield information recorded on the front sheet.

DONOR INFORMATION FOR LEUKAPHERESIS
BY HAEMONETICS INTERRUPTED FLOW CENTRIFUGATION

Following cancer chemotherapy or bone marrow transplantation, patients are often severely depleted of white blood cells which are needed to control infection. Antibiotics can partially control these infections, but replacement of white blood cells from healthy donors is an additional help. The process of obtaining white blood cells from donors is called leukapheresis.

During leukapheresis, units of whole blood are successively removed by a needle from a donor's arm vein and separated by centrifugation into plasma, red blood cells, platelets and white blood cells. The plasma and red blood cells are then returned to the donor through a needle in the other arm. The white blood cells, platelets, and a few red cells are retained for transfusion into the patients. Each donation takes approximately three and one-half hours.

The donor receives physiological saline and three medications during donation: Lidocaine, a local anesthetic; *Citrate,* an anticoagulant used to prevent the donor's blood from clotting while in the machine; *Volex,* a solution necessary for separation of white blood cells from red blood cells.

Prior to donation, each donor's health is evaluated and blood studies are obtained to be certain that the donor can tolerate the procedure with minimal risk and discomfort. During donation, a nurse is present and a physician is available.

Possible risks and discomforts of the procedure include slight pain associated with needle insertion; stiffness in arms, secondary to period of immobilization during donation; tingling around the mouth and nausea due to the citrate; chills caused by the rapid infusion of room temperature blood; bruising at the needle site; and slight allergic reaction and/or slight fluid retention associated with the Volex. Occasionally, a donor will feel faint, but this is uncommon. There is a remote possibility of infection or damage to red blood cells.

If a technical failure (breakage in equipment) occurs, making it impossible to return the red cells and plasma from one bowl filling, the blood loss would be similar to that occurring during donation of whole blood.

If any untoward symptoms are experienced during the 24 hours following donation, they should be reported to the leukapheresis director.

The benefits of a leukapheresis are not direct — the procedure aids not the donor, but the patients receiving the blood products. The need is great and each donation is appreciated.

The staff of this unit is eager to answer any questions the donor may have. A donor is free to withdraw from the program, at any time, for whatever reason.

I have read and discussed the above information with the personnel of the blood products program at the Johns Hopkins Oncology Center. I am willing to donate white blood cells and platelets and receive the medications mentioned above.

Donor Signature: ____

Witness: ____

Date: ____

NOTE: EAT breakfast and/or lunch before donating.
      Do not take aspirin for 48 hours before donation.

May, 1979

Fig 6. — Leukapheresis donor informed consent

DONOR NAME _______________________________

SOCIAL SECURITY NO. _______________________

HLA TYPING _______________________________

BIRTHDATE _______________________________

DATE							
	SCREEN	PRE	POST	PRE	POST	PRE	POST
HCT							
WBC							
PLATELET COUNT							
HEIGHT							
WEIGHT							
HBsAg RIA							
BLOOD GROUP							
BOWL SIZE							
MACHINE #							
NO. OF PASSES							
DONOR ARM							
RECIPIENT							
UNIT #							
YIELD:LEUKOCYTE PROD. WBC							
GRAN.							
PLAT.							
PLATELET PROD. PLAT. II							
PLAT. I OR IA							
PLAT IB							
NURSE/TECHNICIAN							

May 1979

Fig 7. — Front sheet of hemapheresis donor chart

The run sheet contains all of the information about the donation procedure (Fig 8):

1. Donor: height, weight, name, social security number
2. Run: solution volumes, time, flow rate, number of passes, volume processed
3. Vital signs
4. Hematology data
5. Yield information: yields, volume, etc.
6. Quality control data for harnesses, bowls and machines

The run sheets are collected in a series of notebooks to allow assessment of machines, software, and personnel as related to cell yields.

The white cells are issued with the transfusion special chart attached. The special chart is printed on NCR paper so that one copy can be kept in the patient's chart as a transfusion record, and the original can be sent back to the pheresis unit (Fig 9).

Product inventory and quality control data on all inventory are recorded in logs. A malfunction log has been created to document nonstandard performance of software and machine.

Conclusion

This chapter has outlined the design and function of one hospital-based pheresis unit. Other institutions have taken different approaches, depending on the services required and their preexisting resources. Whatever system is utilized, it is important to carefully analyze the components required to assure absolute donor and/or patient safety. The standards for transfusion practice of the Federal Government, the American Red Cross, and the American Association of Blood Banks are a sound basis. However, hemapheresis is a complicated, invasive clinical procedure and the organizational structure of a hemapheresis unit should take that into consideration. This is particularly important when clinical requirements for components and procedures exert pressure for expansion and there is not a large base of historical data on which to structure this growth.

Things to consider in setting up a hemapheresis center:

1. Identify the clinical need for pheresis services, establish utilization criteria and estimates with the users.
2. Develop a method of daily communication for planning and for transfusion responses.
3. Decide on lead time for special requests.
4. Establish the necessary support systems and define their role.
5. Train staff well.

LEUKAPHERESIS

DATE _______________________________   UNIT NO. _______________________________

DONOR _______________________________   SOCIAL SECURITY NO. _______________________

AGE ________   SEX ______   HT. ______   WT. ______   ABO TYPE _______________

BOWL SIZE _______________   NO. OF PASSES ________   FLOW RATE _______________cc/min.

RECIPIENT _______________________   HX. NO. _______________________________

1 Or 2 ARM _______________   TIME START _______________   TIME STOP __________

VOL. NSS _______________   VOLEX _______________   CONC. NA CITRATE ________

     HCT.   WBC   % POLYS   PLATELETS   TOT. PROT.   ALB.

Before _____%   _______________   _______________   _______________   _______________

After _____%   _______________   _______________

TEMP. __________   PULSE _______________   BLOOD PRESSURE _______________

PRE. TOT. BLD. VOL. (ml.) __________   PRE CIRC. WBC (10^9) _______________

VOL. BLD. PROC. (ml.) _______________   WBC/ml. YIELD _______________

AVG. EXTRA CORP. CRC. (ml.) ________   WBC/liter BLD. PROC. _______________

AVG. EXTRA CORP. CRC. (1%) ________   WBC % EFFICIENCY _______________

PRE CIRC. GRAN. (10^9) _______________   PRE CIRC. PLAT. (10^{11}) _______________

GRAN./ml. YIELD _______________   PLAT./ml. YIELD _______________

GRAN. LITER BLD. PROC. _______________   PLAT./liter BLD. PROC. _______________

      PLAT. % EFFICIENCY _______________

WBC PROD. TOT. WBC _______________   TOTAL GRAN. _______________

WBC PROD. TOT. PLATS. _______________

PLAT. PROD. II _______________

PLAT. PROD. I _______________

LOT NO.   EXP. DATE   VOL. WBC ________ ml.   PLATS. PI ________ ml.

BOWL _______________   PLATS. PII ________ ml.

HARNESS _______________   HCT. WBC. ________ %   RBC/WBC ________ ml.

VOLEX _______________   MACHINE _______________

NA CITRATE _______________   Nurse/Technician _______________

FILTER _______________

May 1979

Fig 8. — Leukapheresis run sheet

WHITE BLOOD CELL TRANSFUSION SPECIAL CHART

UNIT   #__________ DATE _______________

RECIPIENT: _____________________________

HOSPITAL NO. ___________________________

INFUSION STARTED AT: _______________ P.M.

TIME DURING INFUSION	BAG #	TEMP	PULSE	BP	RESP	COMMENT
START						
30 min.						
60 min.						
90 min.						
120 min.						
150 min.						
180 min.						
210 min.						

INFUSION TERMINATED AT:_______________ P.M.   TERMINATE PREMATURELY:____YES ____NO

WHY: ____

____

MEDICATION AND EFFECT: ____

____

REACTIONS TO TRANSFUSION: ____YES ____NO

	DURING (Time)	IMMEDIATELY AFTER	DELAYED (Time)
CHILLS			
TACHYPNEA			
CHEST PRESSURE			
FEVER			
BP INCREASE/DECREASE			
SENORIUM			
NAUSEA/VOMITING			
RASH			
ANAPHYLAXIS			
OTHER			

Return white copy to Hemapheresis,
retain yellow copy for your files.

May 1979

Fig 9. — Leukotransfusion special chart

6. Design work so that staff does not spend all day, every day running a machine.
7. Provide time for continuing education.
8. Contact other pheresis units for technical assistance and moral support.

Remember that proper planning and a contented staff will result in a smooth-running productive pheresis unit.

Acknowledgement

I wish to express thanks to Dr. Hayden G. Braine, Charlene V. Jackson, RN, and William J. Ward Jr, for their support and technical assistance.

Chapter 2

ORGANIZATION OF A PHERESIS PROGRAM IN A REGIONAL BLOOD CENTER

Margaret C. McElligott, SBB(ASCP)

Introduction

A REGIONAL BLOOD center should offer a comprehensive program of blood products, immunohematology consultation and specialized laboratory services. As a total supplier of all of the blood banking needs for patients in the hospitals served, the blood center must have the resources (staff, equipment, special laboratories, etc) to provide single-donor platelet and granulocyte concentrates when needed. By providing a centralized shared service, the regional blood center is able to avoid duplication of fixed costs and is able to provide a single fully-utilized service as opposed to a few partially-utilized services in the hospitals. The central concentration of professional knowledge and experience, technical expertise and sophisticated equipment allows the distribution of the most effective therapy available to patients in hospitals of all sizes and types.

Appropriate planning and staffing will allow the regional blood center to overcome the difficulty in assessing candidates for single-donor products in nearby hospitals. Information must be gathered in phone conversations with the attending physicians, consulting hematologist and laboratory personnel, realizing that there is no real substitute for having followed a patient for a period of time and having examined him. When the clinical data are inadequate, it is necessary for the blood center physician to visit the patient. Separation of the collection facility from the transfusion facility makes follow-up difficult, but because it is so necessary, the blood center must provide the mechanism for evaluating each transfusion provided.

The Blood Center of Southeastern Wisconsin (BC), formerly known as the Milwaukee Blood Center, is a regional blood center serving 34 hospitals in a six county area. 95,000 units of whole blood were collected in 1978. There are approximately 200 full-time employees involved both in the operation of the Blood Center and in research activities. The medical staff consists of four physicians, all with academic appointments to the Medical College of Wisconsin.

In 1978, 967 pheresis procedures were performed using three Haemonetics Model 30 cell separators. Of these, 588 were plateletpheresis, 343 were leukapheresis, and 36 were therapeutic procedures. All single-donor platelet concentrates made at the Blood Center of Southeastern Wisconsin are HLA–matched. Single-donor platelet concentrates are transfused only to patients who have been demonstrated to be refractory to pools of fresh random donor platelets.

Staffing

The staffing of a pheresis department presents some unique problems. The demand for pheresis products is neither consistent nor predictable. Products made with current cell separation equipment have a limited storage period, so it is not feasible to stock platelet and white cell concentrates during slack periods. In addition, the precision with which platelet donors are matched to each patient requires selection of a suitable donor immediately prior to transfusion. Frozen storage of platelets may alter this situation in the future. The platelets from donors homozygous at either the HLA-A or -B locus, or from patients in remission, can be stored for future use. Most of the equipment for freezing is available in regional blood centers.

The problems of staffing for occasions when the demand for many platelet and granulocyte transfusion is acute have been considered in the staffing of our pheresis department. Work schedules have been chosen to make pheresis donation convenient for unrelated volunteer donors. Platelet and white cell concentrates are available seven days per week for patients in our region. The department is staffed from 7:30 a.m. to 6:00 p.m. Monday through Friday, and from 9:00 a.m. to 3:00 p.m. on Saturdays. This is done without scheduling overtime hours. Procedures done outside regularly scheduled hours are performed by the full-time staff member on call for that week.

The staff of our Special Pheresis Department consists of the following: the Transfusion Coordinator (TC), who coordinates all resources necessary for transfusion of histocompatible single-donor platelets and granulocytes; four physicians available for consultation in selection of donors and patients for special pheresis products; the supervisor of the Special Pheresis Department; a registered nurse, who is responsible for the operation of the department; and three full-time and one part-time cytopheresis technicians. A clerk handles all routine paper work and filing. Two donor callers, partially responsible to the pheresis department, are available from 9:00 a.m. to 7:00 p.m. weekdays, and from 9:00 a.m. to 2:00 p.m. Saturdays.

Machine usage has been increased and overtime decreased by staggering the work hours of our three full-time technicians. The shifts are

7:00 a.m.-3:30 p.m.; 8:00 a.m.-4:30 p.m.; and 9:30 a.m.-6:00 p.m. Using this schedule, we have been able to perform more procedures each day, to provide breaks and lunch hours, and to allow individuals to donate either before or after work.

Composition of Staff

Our full-time cytopheresis staff consists of two registered nurses and two technicians. At the Blood Center, technicians (non-RN's) perform all routine phlebotomies. In the donor room, these individuals develop good rapport with the donors and handle reactions well. Lay individuals were among the first to learn the pheresis procedure at the BC. Our pheresis technicians have always worked under the supervision of an RN. In view of our six-year experience using a staff of both RN's and technicians, it does not appear to be necessary to employ RN's exclusively in a pheresis unit. By utilizing a combined RN and lay person staff, a cost saving (salaries) can be obtained with no reduction in donor safety.

The pheresis staff is entirely separate from the donor room staff. Using the Haemonetics Model 30, the number of cells collected is entirely dependent on the operator's observations and responses. These skills improve with everyday operation of the machine, so a more consistent product is achieved by a separate pheresis staff. We also avoid the retraining which may be necessary when a rotating staff is utilized.

Transfusion Coordinator

Many resources must be coordinated in a short period of time to provide single-donor platelets and granulocytes. When single-donor products were first made available by BC, the Associate Medical Director was responsible for this coordination. As the demand grew, this function became extremely time-consuming, and a decision was made to hire and train a lay person with a background in biology, nursing, or medical technology to coordinate the transfusion of pheresis products.

The major responsibility of the Transfusion Coordinator (TC) is the coordination of resources, both within the Blood Center (Table 1) and outside of it (Table 2). The resources include: (1) HLA- and ABO-typed on-call donor pool, (2) communication between the BC, the attending physician, and the consulting hematologist, (3) communication between the BC and the transfusion service at the hospital in which the patient is being treated, (4) evaluation of the patient as a potential recipient of our product, (5) selection of donors in best-match order, (6) provision for HLA typing of this recipient, (7) facilitation of cytopheresis scheduling and product processing, (8) delivery of the product,

(9) retrieval and storage of data, and (10) planning of research and data analysis.

Since the activities of many people must be directed to efficiently transfuse histocompatible platelets or white cells, it is essential to have one person coordinate these diverse functions and take the responsibility for insuring that all steps in the process are carried out. In order to coordinate these functions effectively, an understanding of certain principles of transfusion therapy, transplantation immunology, data processing, pheresis technology, and donor recruitment are necessary. It is also essential to be able to communicate effectively with hospitals, physicians, and the other departments of the blood center.

All orders for matched granulocytes or platelets are referred to the Transfusion Coordinator, and the TC contacts the attending physician

---

Table 1. — Blood Center Personnel Involved in Providing Pheresis Products

1. Physician
2. Transfusion Coordinator
3. Supervisor, Special Pheresis Section
4. Supervisor, Tissue Typing Laboratory
5. Director, Tissue Typing Laboratory
6. Clerk, Special Pheresis Section
7. Computer Center
8. Donor Calling Personnel
9. Special Pheresis Technologists
10. Order Department
11. Delivery Department
12. Accounting Department
13. Processing Department

---

and hematologist. Clinical and laboratory data are obtained and evaluated by the TC and, if necessary, the blood center physician, to determine the suitability of the product requested. Arrangements are made with the clinician to procure the necessary blood samples for HLA typing and crossmatching.

The supervisor of the Tissue Typing Laboratory is contacted to ensure prompt attention to the sample for tissue typing. An HLA type usually can be obtained within five hours. With the patient's HLA type, a list of best-matched donors is generated from the HLA- and ABO-typed on-call donor pool. The Computer Center at the Medical College of Wisconsin provides lists of compatible donors for each patient, in best-matched order, as well as a master file of all tissue-typed donors, sorted by their HLA types. From this list, the donor-calling department contacts prospective donors. The Special Pheresis Department is notified of the scheduling of a donor, and preparations are made for drawing this donor. The donation takes place, during which donor samples are tested for hepatitis (short incubation) and syphilis by the Blood Center Processing Laboratory. If granulocytes are being collected, a red cell cross-match is completed by the BC Transfusion Service. Platelet donation requires approximately two hours and white cell donation, about three hours. All testing can be completed during that time. When the platelet unit has been approved for transfusion, it is relayed to the order department, which supplies transportation to the hospital. When the patient is out of town, this process is complicated by having to schedule donors to fit airline schedules. Billing arrangements must be set up in conjunction with the accounting department.

While the procedure and testing are being performed at the Blood Center, contact is maintained with the hospital which is to receive the product. The blood bank, nursing service, and physicians are advised

---

Table 2. — Personnel Involved in Transfusing Pheresis Products

1. Attending Physician and/or House Staff
2. Hematologist
3. Pathologist
4. 'Blood Bank
5. Hematology Laboratory
6. Nursing Staff
7. Hospital Accounting Department
8. Airlines
9. Patient
10. Donors

---

of the time that the product will be available, and any remaining questions are answered.

The most important of all resources in this process is, of course, the donors. Without their willingness to make personal sacrifice and come in on short notice, it would be impossible to support patients requiring matched platelets or granulocytes. We often can provide platelet and granulocyte transfusions the same day they are ordered.

Coordination of histocompatible blood products does not end with the transfusion of the platelets or white cells. Evaluation of transfusion success on a regular basis enables us to select effective donors for subsequent transfusions. Once the transfusion has been administered, the TC is responsible for collection of data on each transfusion, and for analyzing the data. To assist in collecting data for the analysis of every transfusion, forms are provided with each transfusion (Fig 1). If the completed forms are not returned within a reasonable period of time,

THIS SHEET MUST ACCOMPANY PLATELETS TO HOSPITAL.

Please complete this form and return to: **Mrs. Margaret McElligott**
Transfusion Coordinator
Milwaukee Blood Center, Inc.
1701 West Wisconsin Avenue
Milwaukee, Wisconsin 53233

IN ORDER TO SUCCESSFULLY CHOOSE HLA-MATCHED DONORS FOR PATIENTS REFRACTORY TO RANDOM PLATELETS, WE MUST HAVE THE FOLLOWING INFORMATION:

MPT#___________ Date___________ Patient Name_______________________________

Age___________ Sex___________ Weight_______ Hospital_______________________

Physician caring for patient____

Diagnosis_________________________________ Is the patient infected?_________

Is the patient septic?____

Is the patient being given antibiotics?_______ Which?___________________

Is the patient taking quinine, quinidine, thiazides, dilantin, or any drug associated with thrombocytopenia?_________ Which ones?___________________________

Is there evidence of DIC?__________ List________________________________

Does the patient have splenomegaly?_____ Has the patient had a spleen scan?_______

Does the patient have petechiae?_______ Is he/she bleeding?_____ Where?_________

Splenectomy?___________________________ Antihistamines?___________________

Any other blood products within 24 hours of HLA-matched platelets?_____________

TRANSFUSION DATA

We *must* have the platelet counts and temperature pre-transfusion, 1 hour post and 24 hours post transfusion.

	Pre Tx.	1 Hour	24 Hours
PLATELET COUNT			
TEMPERATURE			

Comments on response and clinical situation:_______________________________

____

____

Fig 1. — Platelet transfusion data form

or are returned without all of the necessary data, the physician is contacted to obtain the missing information. Weekly meetings are held to discuss each platelet transfusion, and plans are made to improve results of future transfusions.

Pheresis Donors

The Blood Center of Southeastern Wisconsin, like most regional blood centers, operates under the philosophy that providing blood products is the responsibility of the entire community. This philosophy is carried out in our pheresis program. Our donors are volunteer, nonrelated individuals. The majority of patients refractory to random-donor platelets can be successfully transfused with platelets from nonrelated donors who are close HLA matches.[1]

The Blood Center of Southeastern Wisconsin has a list of 9,400 persons who have volunteered to donate whole blood and blood components when there is a specific need for blood of their type (On-Call-Donors). More than 8,800 of these donors have been HLA-typed. Permission for detailed typing of blood, and storage of donor information is obtained whenever a donation is made.

Utilizing perfect HLA matches and crossreacting matches of donor and recipient, an average of 400 compatible donors are available for each patient. The number of HLA-compatible donors available for each patient ranges from 12 to 1,410.

In 1978, the Blood Center of Southeastern Wisconsin provided 931 pheresis products, using a total of 583 donors. The most frequently used donor was drawn eight times in that period. Most of the donors were pheresed only once. It is evident that the burden of providing matched platelet and granulocyte support need not rest on family members and friends of the patient, or on a few reliable volunteer or paid donors. Because none of our donors are pheresed frequently, we may, in addition, reduce the chance of presently unknown long-term side effects of pheresis donation.

Pheresis donors are encouraged to continue donating whole blood. With only 4% of the nation's eligible donors giving blood, and the need for blood increasing every year, it is important to encourage frequent donations.

An attempt is made to utilize many different donors as pheresis donors. It is easier to recruit when donors can be assured that they will not be asked to donate every week. This strategy has also helped the BC to maintain good relations with the donors' employers. A large pool of HLA-typed individuals also provide a better selection of donors for each patient.

The utilization of nonrelated donors is desirable in several respects: (1) additional stress is not put on the patient and his family by making them responsible for procuring donors, and a family member reluctant to be pheresed is not made to feel guilty, or that the patient's life has been jeopardized; (2) patients without family and friends eligible for pheresis are not denied these products; (3) for some patients, better HLA matches are available in the nonrelated donor pool than in their families; and (4) pheresis of nonrelated donors can be carried out on the same professional level as whole blood donations — the highly emotional element involved when family members act as donors is absent.

Recruitment of Donors

Blood donors, not pheresis donors, are recruited by the Blood Center of Southeastern Wisconsin. Whole-blood donors are given the opportunity to become "On-Call Donors." On-Call Donors agree to be contacted when blood or blood components of their specific type is needed. These donors are HLA-typed and serve as both whole-blood and pheresis donors.

Many of our On-Call Donors are not aware of the pheresis program until they are contacted for a donation for a specific patient. The contact is made by a donor caller. The caller tells the donor that his tissue type matches that of a patient in need of platelets (or granulocytes). The donor then hears an explanation of the procedure and is asked if he is interested. A series of questions is asked to determine his eligibility. The donor is never made to feel that he is the only donor suitable for that patient.

This approach to recruiting has been quite successful. Approximately 75% of the donors who hear the explanation of the procedure express a willingness to participate. An advantage of this system is that every first-time pheresis donor has had the experience of donating whole blood in the routine fashion at least once.

Storage and Retrieval of Donor Data

With almost 9,000 available donors, computerized storage and retrieval of donor data is a necessity. Each donor's name, address, phone number, ABO type, Rh type, HLA type, and eligibility date are part of the information entered into the computer. A printout of all On-Call Donors, sorted by HLA type, is obtained monthly. At any time, a patient's HLA type can be submitted to the computer and a list of matched donors will be printed, ranked in the order of best match to worst match. If needed, the computer will generate a list of donors who are both HLA- and

ABO-compatible with the patient. From this individualized patient print-out, a list of the best donors for the patient is generated by the TC. This list is utilized by our donor callers in procuring suitable donors for the patient.

Informed Consent

Each time a donor gives whole blood, consent is obtained for detailed typing of his blood and for storage of pertinent data. Before he is cytopheresed, the procedure and possible side effects are explained by the cytopheresis technician. A consent form must be signed before the procedure can be initiated.

Communication With Physician and Follow-Up
of the Transfusion

The regional blood center becomes a consultant in patient care when matched platelets or granulocytes are requested. The regional center must determine whether the product requested is appropriate.[2] If the product seems to be appropriate, and a transfusion is given, the result must be evaluated by the regional center to help in the selection of blood products for that patient in the future. Communication between the regional blood center and the physician caring for the patient is essential in providing good care for that patient.

When a hospital requests matched platelets or granulocytes from the BC, the attending physician and/or consulting hematologist are contacted by the TC. The patient's clinical history, transfusion history, evidence of infections, spleen size, antibiotics, chemotherapy, bone marrow status, laboratory test results, and other necessary data are obtained (Fig 2). Potential recipients of granulocytes are seen by a BC physician and the TC. The suitability of the requested product is evaluated by the TC. Arrangements are made with the hospital physician to obtain necessary blood samples, and he is told when to expect the product, and what laboratory work is required for follow-up. If the use of the pheresis product does not meet established criteria, the ordering physician is contacted by a BC physician to discuss the request.

All requests for pheresis products are examined closely to ensure that the patient receives the proper blood component. This is important in protecting the patient's health and in cost containment. Matched platelets and granulocytes are quite costly. In addition, these products, like all blood products, are not without risk. Prudent use of a limited resource, our donors, must also be considered.

All patients transfused with platelets must have platelet counts per-

MATCHED PLATELET AND WHITE CELL TRANSFUSIONS

Date of Call: ____

Physician caring for patient: _____________________ Physician phone: __________

Name of patient: ____________________________ Weight: ____ Age: ____ Race: ____

Hospital: ____________________________________ Room: ____ ABO-Rh: ____

Diagnosis: ____

    Does the patient have splenomegaly? ____ Has the patient had a splenectomy? ____

    Is the patient infected? _______________ Is the patient septic? _____________

    Is the patient refractory to random platelets? ____ Is the patient on antibiotics? ____

    What antibiotics? ______________________________________

    Is there mucous membrane bleeding? ____ Does the patient have petechiae? ____

    Has the patient received chemotherapy? _______ How many courses? _________

        What drugs? _______________________________________

        When was chemotherapy completed? _______________________

        Has the patient gone into remission? ____ How many times? ________

    Have blood cultures been done? _______ When? ________________________

        Results: ____

    Has a bone marrow been done? _______ When? _________________________

        Results: ____

    Transfusion History: ___________________________________

____

____

____

Will send: Bill to & Ship to: _______

    10 ml Hep or ACD _______________________________________

    10 ml clot ____

    (10 ml clot to Ref.) _____________________________________

    Computer or Lab printout: _________________________________

        of plt cts ____

        WBC cts ____

        differentials _______________________________________

        any other lab work __________________________________

    Xerox of discharge or clinical summary ______________________

    Xerox of medication schedule for ___________________________

        chemotherapy & antibiotics of current admission _____________

Fig 2. — Patient data form

formed immediately prior to transfusion, one hour after the transfusion has been completed, and 24 hours following the transfusion. Vital signs must be recorded during the transfusion, as well as any symptoms of a reaction. This information, plus some clinical information, are recorded on a form that accompanies each platelet transfusion (Fig 1). These forms are to be returned to the TC within 48 hours of the transfusion. If the forms are not returned, the patient's physician is contacted by the TC. Contact is maintained until the results are received. Weekly meetings involving BC physicians, Transfusion Coordinator, the director of the HLA Laboratory, supervisor of the HLA Laboratory and the supervisor of the Special Pheresis Department are held to evaluate these transfusions and to determine the reason for success or failure. A list of potentially-effective donors for subsequent transfusions is prepared at each meeting. The patient benefits directly from prompt follow-up of these transfusions.

Granulocyte transfusions are still in a developmental stage. The best way to evaluate these transfusions has not been determined. More research must be done to determine which patients should receive granulocyte transfusions and how to evaluate their effectiveness.

Summary

Single-donor pheresis products should not be distributed indiscriminately. Available donors are a limited resource and must be used judiciously. Pheresis platelets are more expensive than those produced from units of whole blood. HLA-matched platelets should be reserved for patients refractory to random-donor platelets. There are also certain risks associated with the transfusion of platelets and granulocytes which must be weighed against possible benefit to the recipient.

The regional blood center is part of the health care delivery system. By providing blood products, immunohematology consultation, specialized laboratory services and educational programs, the regional blood center improves the quality of patient care in the community.

References

1. Duquesnoy RJ: Donor selection in platelet transfusion therapy of alloimmunized thrombocytopenic patients, in Greenwalt T (ed): *The Blood Platelet in Transfusion Therapy*. New York, Alan R Liss, Inc, 1978, p 229-244.
2. Harker LA, Slichter SJ: The bleeding time as a screening test for evaluation of platelet function. *N Engl J Med* 287:155-59, 1972.

Chapter 3

DONOR SELECTION FOR PHERESIS DONATION

Alfred J. Katz, MD

MANY OF THE DONOR considerations for a pheresis donation are comparable to those for whole blood donation. In general, those professionally responsible for the donation must assure that the risk to the recipient of the product is minimized, and that the criteria for protection of the donor are met. In addition, through the process of informed consent, the donor must understand and accept the risk of donation.

The benefit of the pheresis product to the recipient, for some products and in some circumstances, may be debated. However, for most patient-recipients, the potential benefit to be gained from the transfusion of the product far outweighs the risks of receiving the transfusion. The benefits include platelet transfusion to treat or prevent life-threatening thrombocytopenic bleeding, and granulocyte transfusion to augment other therapies in serious infection associated with granulocytopenia.

For the donor, the situation may be quite different. Recent studies of platelet- and plasmapheresis donors have documented that the act of donation may be motivated by a need to help others, to achieve a sense of purpose, to respond to pressures from community service groups,[1] or to achieve credit for a nonreplacement fee.[2] The altruistic behavior of the voluntary donor may be an act of giving, as well as an opportunity to receive emotional gratification in fulfillment of important psychological needs.[3] For some donors, the motivation to donate frequently is great, and as for donors of whole blood,[4] may approach Munchausen Syndrome proportions. In return for the gratification of donating, the donor, depending upon the procedure, may be subject to physical risk — some of which may not be well understood at this time. The pheresis procedures being employed widely should be considered experimental; the potential risks to the donor should be evaluated carefully and conservatively, eliminated wherever possible, and where they remain, explained to the donor.

The discussion that follows will consider, in turn, donor medical history criteria, pre- and postpheresis tests on donors, the impact of frequent donations on the donor, the variety of medications to which the donor may be exposed, and the rationale for selection of a family member or nonrelated volunteer matched donor. No attempt will be made to organize this material according to the specific varieties of pheresis procedures, although there are differences which will be recognized. Other contributors to this workshop will review current procedures in more detail.

Medical History Criteria

In general, the health history criteria which are applicable for whole blood donation are relevant for protection of both donor and recipient, and should be applied prior to pheresis donation. Standards for such criteria are widely known.[5] Initial evaluation must also include temperature, blood pressure, pulse, and hemoglobin or hematocrit. For the pheresis donor, there are health history considerations which require special attention.

- Has the prospective donor had an adverse reaction to prior pheresis donation? If so, what was the nature of that reaction? Of concern, for example, would be development of signs of hypersensitivity reaction, possibly in response to a sedimenting agent such as hydroxyethyl starch, to heparin, or to steroids.

- Does the donor have a history of thrombocytopenia or of abnormal bleeding episodes? This question is critical if the procedure requires the use of heparin; an accurate bleeding history may be more important in signaling a problem than are the laboratory screening tests usually performed. Women donors should not receive heparin during menses.

- Is the donor allergic to beef or pork, either of which may be the source of heparin to be infused before and for use during a procedure?

- Does the donor have a history suggestive of fluid retention — independent of, or associated with a previous pheresis donation? Swelling of hands or feet, or puffiness of eyes would be suggestive, and would require careful evaluation for disqualification for a procedure in which steroids and/or hydroxyethyl starch would be used.

- Has the donor had any of a variety of disorders which may be exacerbated by administration of corticosteroids? The list is long, and includes hypertension, duodenal ulcer, diabetes mellitus, and tuberculosis.

- What is the donor's weight? Some pheresis procedures involve a relatively large extracorporeal blood volume during collection. Selection of large donors, or modification of procedure (eg, small volume bowls for intermittent-flow centrifugation) must be made to assure that extracorporeal volume will not be excessive.

- Has the donor taken any medication which may place the donor at greater risk, or which may render the product ineffective? Both results can occur if any one of a vast number of medications containing aspirin have been ingested in the days immediately preceding donation. Aspirin is an antithrombotic agent, whose effect is due to its ability to irreversibly acetylate platelet cyclooxygenase, and thereby, inhibit platelet aggregation.[6,7] Transfusion of "aspirinated" platelets to a severely thrombocytopenic recipient is unlikely to be effective therapy unless one-tenth or more of the circulating platelets are fully functional.[8] For this reason, at least three days should elapse between donation and the time of prior aspirin medication. The effect of aspirin on granulocyte function is less clear. A recent report[9] suggests that, although baseline in vitro function may be normal, granulocytes previously exposed to aspirin will not exhibit increased adherence to nylon fibers in the presence of bacterial products, and may not appear in normal numbers in exudates in experimental peritonitis in mice. Administration of heparin to a donor who has taken aspirin may compound a hemostatic defect. The *Standards*[5] of the American Association of Blood Banks note that: "Leukapheresis donors who have ingested aspirin or aspirin-containing medication within 48 hours of a procedure requiring heparinization should have a normal bleeding time at the time of the procedure."

Should any problems be noted in any of the above areas, they should be referred to a physician who is knowledgeable in the areas of pheresis. If an exception to standard criteria is made, and this exception entails further risk to the donor, appropriate explanation must be made and consent must be received. In general, exception is made only when the cells from a selected donor are of special value for a specific recipient.

Laboratory Tests for Donors

In order to help assure donor safety, hemoglobin or hematocrit and serum protein should be measured prior to each procedure. In addition, donor platelet concentration should not be less than $150,000/\mu l$; a post-pheresis platelet count from a prior procedure acceptably provides this assurance. For donors undergoing leukapheresis, predonation white cell count and differential should be obtained for documentation, and for correlation with the yield of product obtained. A partial thromboplastin time should be obtained prior to heparin administration. A serum protein electropheresis should be obtained every four months if a donor is undergoing regular, eg, biweekly, pheresis procedures.

Frequency of Donation

Many factors influence the frequency of pheresis donation by a given individual, some psychologic, some logistic, and some physiologic. In practice, within medically-acceptable limits, some donors may undergo pheresis a number of times within a week, while others may be called to donate only one or two times per year. A service which calls upon family-member donors is likely to use those donors more frequently and for a few weeks at a time. A patient who requires products from selected, matched donors may require frequent donations from a small number of individuals. Both family members and volunteers may be motivated to donate frequently, although the former group, more so. And, although members of both groups can be presumed to be motivated by a desire to help, members of both may become psychologically burdened by the dependence of a patient upon the specific pheresis donation.

Time in which to donate may be another consideration. Many pheresis programs have recognized this and have organized collection hours to suit the convenience of donors much more than to fit usual staff working hours. Also, it may not be possible to gain access to donor veins which have been punctured repeatedly.

Of major concern in this workshop are the physiologic impacts of donation and their implication for frequency of donation. The extent of plasma removal may be a consideration, depending upon the procedure and the specific technic used. Loss of plasma may be minimal in filtration leukapheresis, but may be as much as 300-500 ml using intermittent-flow centrifugation (IFC) and a red cell sedimenting agent. Plasma removal and recumbency during donation lead to immediate and relatively transient dilutional and postural changes.[10] Immediately following plateletpheresis, our donors showed a 17% decrease in total serum protein concentration.[11] Those donating and losing plasma frequently are at potential risk of protein — including immunoglobulin — depletion. For these reasons, limits of 1,000 ml per seven days, and 15 liters per year (World Health Organization) have been established for plasma removal from an individual, and serum protein electrophoresis is indicated as outlined above.

A number of reports have shown that the yield of platelets from plateletpheresis exceeds the decrease in the number of platelets circulating in the donor.[12-14] The finding suggests mobilization of platelets during the procedure, primarily from the splenic pool.[13,15] Overall, there is about a 30% decrease in concentration of circulating platelets during an IFC procedure; the initial concentration is reestablished in three days following a single procedure. Safe, consecutive-day removal of platelets by quadruple plateletpheresis pack has been reported;[16] mean day-to-day decrease in count was 13% (range +56 to −54%). Of all donor variables, platelet count will be most closely correlated with platelet yield.

Removal of platelets in the usual plateletpheresis procedures does not appear to be a major stimulus to thrombopoeisis. It seems reasonable, therefore, to limit platelet loss to once in three days, although plateletpheresis can safely be performed more frequently if a single donor's cells are particularly needed. Most importantly, the donor's platelet count must be monitored to assure that the donor is not placed at risk from thrombocytopenia. Platelet counts will be decreased also during continuous-flow leukapheresis and filtration leukapheresis,[17] although the latter procedure has been reported to have been performed as often as eight times in ten days without severe donor thrombocytopenia.

Circulating leukocyte and granulocyte counts are not decreased by the variety of platelet and leukapheresis in common practice, even when procedures are repeated frequently on the same donor.[17] Immediate-post-pheresis reports of change have included (1) a decrease of 600 granulocytes/μl following continuous-flow leukapheresis,[17] and (2) an increase of 610 granulocytes/μl following intermittent-flow plateletpheresis.[14] Granulocyte counts are, on average, increased following filtration leukapheresis,[17] although the extent of increase may be influenced by steroids commonly given prior to the procedure.[18] Donors develop neutropenia within 10 to 20 minutes of the start of the filtration procedure,[18,19] a finding associated temporally with,[20] and attributable to complement activation. The changes in granulocyte counts during, and immediately after pheresis donation do not limit the frequency of donation by an individual.

In the course of plateletpheresis by intermittent-flow centrifugation $2\text{-}5 \times 10^9$ lymphocytes may be removed.[14,22] Study of two donors during long-term plateletpheresis suggests that normal numbers of lymphocytes continue to circulate.[23] Donors who regularly participate in plateletpheresis do not appear to develop overt immunologic disorders which may be associated with loss of lymphocytes. However, subclinical, low-frequency, or long-term adverse effects should be considered and investigated.

During pheresis procedures, erythrocytes are lost to the donor through the cell collection process and mixture with the desired product, through loss in the collection system, and through blood samples for testing for donor and product safety and for experimental purpose. Estimates of red cell loss range from 36 to 82 ml of cells during continuous-flow leukapheresis, and 67 ml of cells during filtration leukapheresis.[17] Red cell loss may be higher in intermittent-flow leukapheresis and, for all of these procedures, it is important to estimate red cell loss for each donor. Total loss of red cells per year, through pheresis and whole blood donation, should be no greater than the equivalent of 1,800-1,980 ml of whole blood. Donation of 450 ml of whole blood requires deferral for eight weeks, unless all other criteria for donation have been met and specific approval is granted by a qualified physician.

In summary, loss of plasma, platelets, and red cells may occur to significant extent during a pheresis procedure. The extent of loss of these components will effect the frequency with which an individual may donate. Exceptions to guidelines must be evaluated by a qualified physician.

Effects of Medications on Donor Selection

Heparin is the anticoagulant required for filtration leukapheresis, and it has been used in other collection procedures as well. Its clinical use has been reviewed recently.[24] Heparin is widespread in animal tissues, and its main sources for pharmaceutical preparations are beef lung and porcine intestinal mucosa. It functions as an anticoagulant by greatly accelerating the rate at which antithrombin III neutralizes proteolytic activity in the coagulation sequence. Potential adverse effects include bleeding, allergic reactions, and thrombocytopenia; the latter perhaps related to antiplatelet antibody dependent upon heparin.

Doses used in filtration leukapheresis have been reported to vary greatly,[25] from 3,500 to 45,000 units per collection procedure, with a median of 15,000 units. It is administered by bolus before and during the procedure; by continuous addition to blood as it is drawn from the donor during the procedure; and in various combinations of the two approaches. There apparently is little current agreement on the optimum or standard dose and route of administration, and a service beginning to use filtration leukapheresis is advised to follow the manufacturer's instructions. Use of heparin requires that the prospective donor be carefully queried about bleeding history, menses, history of aspirin ingestion, allergy to beef or pork, and previous adverse reaction during a pheresis procedure.

Protamine sulfate may be used at the end of the procedure to neutralize residual heparin. Alternatively, donors may be asked to remain at the pheresis site for up to a few hours to further decrease the remote risk of accident or adverse reaction while anticoagulated. Protamines are strongly basic proteins, found in the sperm of salmon and other fish. Bolus infusion may cause hypotension, bradycardia, dyspnea, flushing, and feeling of warmth. If protamine is to be used, donors must be asked about prior adverse reaction to protamine administration.

Citrate, as sodium citrate, ACD-A or ACD-B, is the other widely used anticoagulant for pheresis procedures. Citrate ions anticoagulate by chelating divalent cations necessary for the coagulation process, and donor symptoms, such as paresthesias, are related to the concentration of citrate, the cumulative citrate dose, and the rate of citrate administration.[26,27] A number of studies have reported the effects of citrate on ionized calcium and donor ECG,[27-29] and authors generally have recommended the use of 2% citrate, ACD-B, diluted ACD-A, or other solutions[30] to decrease donor symptoms and signs of hypocalcemia. ACD-B has also been reported to give higher yields of platelets than ACD-A or 2% citrate.[26] The implication for donor selection is to emphasize the need to obtain an accurate history of cardiac disease and particularly arrhythmia, and for careful evaluation of pulse.

Corticosteroids have been administered to potential donors of granulocytes, primarily in order to increase the circulating number of granulocytes and, thereby, to increase the yield of these cells in the final product. Dexamethasone, whether administered orally or intravenously, in doses of 4-8 mgm/m^2, will produce maximum granulocytosis, associated with lymphopenia, 4-6 hours postadministration.[31] Oral prednisone will produce similar effects 4-6 hours after administration, and the effects last for 24-36 hours.[32] Enhancement of the effect can be achieved by divided doses of dexamethasone, 3 mgm/m^2 p.o. 12 and 3 hours prior to the leukapheresis procedure.[33]

These observations suggest that dexamethasone administered immediately before a procedure will not have time to exert maximal effect on the number of circulating granulocytes. That conclusion is supported by absence of increase in yield by filtration leukapheresis in two studies,[32,34] although some increase was seen in a third.[35] In the latter, use of intravenous dexamethasone was also associated with improved posttransfusion increments in recipients, improved granulocyte morphology, and decreased incidence of donor and recipient adverse reactions.

Increases in yield specifically related to steroid administration hours in advance of the procedure have been reported for filtration,[32] continuous-flow[32,36] and intermittent-flow[37] procedures. The effects of steroids on granulocyte function have been studied[38-41] and reviewed.[42] Although there are differences in methodology, and although some adverse effects have been reported, at this time there is no reason to conclude that steroids adversely effect the clinical utility of granulocyte transfusion, nor do they appear to significantly effect platelet function.[43,44]

Single-dose administration of steroids in experimental setting[31] was associated with headache, fever, tiredness, sweating, and change in mood and performance. Other potential adverse effects include exacerbation of diabetes mellitus, tuberculosis, ulcers, and hypertension. Donor history should consider these possibilities specifically. Similarly, although single doses of steroids carry little risk, frequent administration may be of greater consequence and requires the establishment of procedural guidelines. One such reported guideline[35] is to limit steroid stimulation to four times per donor, and to no more than twice weekly. On the other hand, corticosteroid pretreatment of donors appears to be effective in decreasing the incidence of abdominal pain in female donors undergoing filtration leukapheresis.[45] The consequence of the two concerns may be to limit the frequency with which individual donors participate in filtration leukapheresis.

Another important adjunct to the collection of granulocytes by centrifugation is the use of a red cell sedimentating agent.[46] Most commonly used is 6% hydroxyethyl starch (HES) in normal saline, to which citrate is added as anticoagulant. Originally, HES was developed as a blood volume expander, and is effective as such because the hydroxyethyl group resists hydrolysis by amylase. Hydroxyethyl starch has been used extensively in centrifugation leukapheresis, and it, or another sedimenting agent, must be used to maximize yields of granulocytes.[36,37,47-51] Reports of adverse effects on donors have been few, and there apparently are no adverse effects on the granulocytes[52,53] and platelets.[53,54] Dextran 110 and 150[55] and Dextran 75,[56] also, have been used successfully as sedimenting agents.

Concerns with the use of HES are related to (a) side effects of fluid retention, particularly if used frequently, (b) anaphylactoid responses, which have been reported following 0.085% of HES infusions,[57] and (c) retention of small amounts of HES in the circulation several months after infusion, with unknown long-term consequences.[58]

Rationale for Selection of Family Member, Random Volunteer, or Matched Volunteer Donor

Single-donor plateletpheresis products may be obtained from random donors to meet inventory needs for platelet concentrates that cannot be met otherwise. Other than theoretically to reduce risk of posttransfusion hepatitis, there is no clear indication to preferentially transfuse a plateletpheresis product to a nonrefractory recipient in lieu of random single-unit concentrates.

Selection of a donor for plateletpheresis becomes necessary when a patient becomes refractory to random platelet concentrates. The most widely available approach to the selection of such a donor is through matching for HLA-A, and B antigens.[59-62] The pool of compatible matches may be extended by consideration of cross-reactive antigens.[63-65] However, for the individual donor-recipient pair, the quality of the HLA match appears to be not as fully predictive of in vivo response as desirable,[65,66] and therefore, empiric platelet crossmatch technics have been evaluated. These have included platelet aggregometry, serotonin release, platelet factor 3 release, and lymphocytotoxicity,[67-70] but there is no consensus that these tests are of value. Platelet immunofluence has been reported to be predictive of in vivo success 93% of the time,[71] and a combination of serotonin release and radioimmune assay for platelet-bound IgG has been reported to have 84% predictive success.[72]

The latter report by Slichter[72] also summarizes experience with family-member and unrelated donors, indicating that successful in vivo results will be achieved 30% of the time with haploidentical family donors, and 68% of the time if A or B grade HLA matches are made with nonrelated donors. One or more compatible donors were found among family members for 44% of alloimmunized recipients. Clearly, family-member donors represent a valuable resource and should be actively recruited on that basis.

The alloimmunized recipient also may require special donor selection for granulocyte transfusion. Lower posttransfusion granulocyte increments may occur if the donor and recipient are mismatched for HLA antigens.[73,74]

Studies in dogs have indicated that animals sensitized to donor antigens prior to being made granulocytopenic have poor increments post-granulocyte transfusion.[75,76] Sensitization was associated also with increased incidence of early death from sepsis in dogs.[76] Tests for anti-leukocyte antibody in human donor-recipient pairs identified such antibody in 52% of recipients, but presence of antibody was not related to granulocyte recovery or incidence of transfusion reaction.[77] It seems likely, therefore, that improved technics for selection of granulocyte donors by typing and crossmatching will be needed.

References

1. Cataldo JF, Cohen E, Morganti JB: Motivation of voluntary plasma-pheresis donors. *Transfusion* 16:375, 1976.

2. Wendlant GMcC, Lichtiger B: A highly specialized and motivated volunteer population: platelet donors. *Transfusion* 17:218, 1977.

3. Szymanski LS, Cushna B, Jackson BCH, et al: Motivation of plateletpheresis donors. *Transfusion* 18:64, 1978.

4. Lefer LG, Rosier RP: Munchausen syndrome: blood bank variety. *JAMA* 239:296, 1978.

5. *Standards for Blood Banks and Transfusion Services,* ed 9. Washington, DC, American Association of Blood Banks, 1978.

6. Roth GJ, Majerus PW. The mechanism of the effect of aspirin on human platelets. I. Acetylation of a particulate fraction protein. *J Clin Invest.* 56:624, 1975.

7. Burch JW, Stanford N, Majerus PW: Inhibition of platelet prostaglandin synthetase by oral aspirin. *J Clin Invest* 61:314, 1978.

8. O'Brien JR: Effects of salicylates on human platelets. *Lancet* 1:1431, 1968.

9. Spagnuolo PJ, Ellner JJ: Salicylate blockade of granulocyte adherence and the inflammatory response to experimental peritonitis. *Blood* 53:1018, 1979.

10. Friedman BA, Schork MA, Alm SK, et al: Plasmapheresis-induced hemodilution and its effects on serum constituents. *Transfusion* 16:155, 1976.

11. Reiss RF, Katz AJ: Statewide support of thrombocytopenic patients with ABO matched single donor platelets. *Transfusion* 16:312, 1976.

12. Szymanski IO, Patti K, Kliman A: Efficacy of the Latham blood processor to perform plateletpheresis. *Transfusion* 13:405, 1973.

13. Katz AJ, Reiss RF, Houx JA: Redistribution of platelets during discontinuous flow platelet pheresis. *Vox Sang* 35:345, 1978.

14. Nusbacher J, Scher ML, MacPherson, JL: Plateletpheresis using the Haemonetics model 30 cell separator. *Vox Sang* 33:9, 1977.

15. Slichter SJ. Efficacy of platelets collected by semi-continuous flow centrifugation (Haemonetics Model 30). *Br J Haematol* 38:131, 1978.

16. Schiffer CA, Buchholz DH, Wiernik PH: Intensive multiunit plateletpheresis of normal donors. *Transfusion* 14:388, 1974.

17. Buchholz DH, Schiffer CA, Wiernik PH, et al: Granulocyte harvest for transfusion: donor response to repeated leukapheresis. *Transfusion* 15:96, 1975.

18. Rubins JM, MacPherson JL, Nusbacher J, et al: Granulocyte kinetics in donors undergoing filtration leukapheresis. *Transfusion* 16:56, 1976.

19. Schiffer CA, Aisner J, Wiernik PH: Transient neutropenia induced by transfusion of blood exposed to nylon fiber filters. *Blood* 45:141, 1975.

20. Nusbacher J, Rosenfeld SI, MacPherson JL, et al: Nylon fiber leukapheresis: associated complement component changes and granulocytopenia. *Blood* 51:359, 1978.

21. Hammerschmidt DE, Craddock PR, McCullough J, et al: Complement activation and pulmonary leukostasis during nylon fiber filtration leukapheresis. *Blood* 51:721, 1978.

22. Genco PV, Katz AJ: Redistribution of lymphocytes during discontinuous flow plateletpheresis. *Blood* 52:298, 1978.

23. Lichtiger B, Trujillo JM, Fischer HE, et al: T and B cell populations in platelet donors. *Tumori* 64:613, 1978.

24. Wessler S, Gitel SN: Heparin: new concepts relevant to clinical use. *Blood* 53:525, 1979.

25. Buchholz DH, Houx JL: Filtration leukapheresis: a survey of current collection and transfusion techniques. *Exp Hematol* 7:1, 1979.

26. Huestis DW, Fletcher JL, White RF, et al: Citrate anticoagulants for plateletpheresis. *Transfusion* 17:151, 1977.

27. Olson PR, Cox C, McCullough J: Laboratory and clinical effects of the infusion of ACD solution during plateletpheresis. *Vox Sang* 33:79, 1977.

28. Ladenson JH, Miller WV, Sherman LA: Relationship of physical symptoms, ECG, free calcium, and other blood chemistries in reinfusion with citrated blood. *Transfusion* 18:670, 1978.

29. Szymanski IO: Ionized calcium during plateletpheresis. *Transfusion* 18:701, 1978.

30. Mishler JM, Janes AW, Lowes B, et al: The utilization of a new strength citrate anticoagulant during centrifugal plateletpheresis. I. Assessment of donor effects. *Brit. J. Haematol* 34:385, 1976.

31. Mishler JM, Emerson PM: Development of neutrophilia by serially increasing doses of dexamethasone. *Brit J Haematol* 36:249, 1977.

32. MacPherson JL, Nusbacher J, Bennett JM: The acquisition of granulocytes by leukapheresis: a comparison of continuous-flow centrifugation and filtration leukapheresis in normal and corticosteroid-stimulated donors. *Transfusion* 16:221, 1976.

33. Winton EF, Vogler WR: Development of a practical oral dexamethasone premedication schedule leading to improved granulocyte yields with the continuous-flow centrifugal blood cell separator. *Blood* 52:249, 1978.

34. Katz AJ, Houx J, Morse EE: Factors affecting the efficiency of filtration leukapheresis. *Transfusion* 17:67, 1977.

35. Higby DJ, Henderson ES, Burnett D, et al: Filtration leukapheresis: effects of donor stimulation with dexamethasone. *Blood* 50:953, 1977.

36. Bearden JD III, Coltman CA Jr, Ratkin GA: Hydroxyethyl starch and prednisone as adjuncts to granulocyte collection. *Transfusion* 17:141, 1977.

37. Sussman LN: Efficient preparation of platelets and granulocytes from single donors, using the cell processor. *Lab Med* 9:21, 1978.

38. Shoji M, Vogler WR: Effects of hydrocortisone on the yield and bactericidal function of granulocytes collected by continuous-flow centrifugation. *Blood* 44:435, 1974.

39. Glasser L, Huestis DW, Jones JF: Functional capabilities of steroid-recruited neutrophils harvested for clinical transfusion. *N Engl J Med* 297:1033, 1977.

40. Steigbigel RT, Baum J, MacPherson JL, et al: Granulocyte bactericidal capacity and chemotaxis as affected by continuous-flow centrifugation and filtration leukapheresis, steroid administration, and storage. *Blood* 52:197, 1978.

41. Clark RAF, Gallin JI, Fauci AS: Effects of in vivo prednisone on in vitro eosinophil and neutrophil adherence and chemotaxis. *Blood* 53:633, 1979.

42. Mishler JM: The effects of corticosteroids on mobilization and function of neutrophils. *Exp Hematol* 5:16, 1977.

43. Thong KL, Mant MJ, Grace MG: Lack of effect of prednisone administration on bleeding time and platelet function of normal subjects. *Brit J Haematol* 38:373, 1978.

44. Lichtenfeld KM, Schiffer CA: The effect of dexamethasone on platelet function. *Transfusion* 19:169, 1979.

45. Wiltbank TB, Nusbacher J, Higby DJ, et al: Abdominal pain in donors during filtration leukapheresis. *Transfusion* 17:159, 1977.

46. Roy AJ, Simmons WB, Franklin A, et al: Hydroxyethyl starch for separation of normal granulocytes. *Fed Proc* 29:424, 1970.

47. McCredie KB, Freireich EJ, Hester JP, et al: Increased granulocyte collection using the blood cell separator and the addition of etiocholanolone and hydroxyethyl starch. *Transfusion* 14:357, 1974.

48. Mishler JM, Higby DJ, Rhomberg W, et al: Hydroxyethyl starch and dexamethasone as an adjunct to leukocyte separation with the IBM blood cell separator. *Transfusion* 14:352, 1974.

49. Mishler JM, Hadlock DC, Fortuny IE, et al: Increased efficiency of leukocyte collection by the addition of hydroxyethyl starch to the continuous-flow centrifuge. *Blood* 44:571, 1974.

50. Huestis DW, White RF, Price MJ, et al: Use of hydroxyethyl starch to improve granulocyte collection in the Latham blood processor. *Transfusion* 15:559, 1975.

51. Mishler JM, Moser AM, Carter JB: The safety of dexamethasone and hydroxyethyl starch in the multiply leukapheresed donor. *Transfusion* 16:170, 1976.

52. Strauss RG, Maguire LC, Koepke JA, et al: Properties of neutrophils collected by discontinuous-flow centrifugation leukapheresis employing hydroxyethyl starch. *Transfusion* 19:192, 1979.

53. Schiffer CA, Aisner J, Schmukler M, et al: The effect of hydroxyethyl starch on in vitro platelet and granulocyte function. *Transfusion* 15:473, 1975.

54. Farrales FB, Belcher C, Summers T, et al: Effect of hydroxyethyl starch on platelet function following granulocyte collection using the continuous flow cell separator. *Transfusion* 17:635, 1977.

55. Lowenthal RM, Park DS: The use of dextran as an adjunct to granulocyte collection with the continuous-flow blood cell separator. *Transfusion* 15:23, 1975.

56. Huestis DW: Use of dextran 75 as a macromolecular agent in centrifugal leukapheresis. *Transfusion* 17:156, 1977.

57. Ring J, Messmer K: Incidence and severity of anaphylactoid reactions to colloid volume substitutes. *Lancet* i:466, 1977.

58. Boon JC, Jesch F, Ring J, et al: Intravascular persistence of hydroxyethyl starch in man. *Eur Surg Res* 8:497, 1976.

59. Yankee RA, Grumet FC, Rogentine GN: Platelet transfusion therapy. The selection of compatible platelet donors for refractory patients by lymphocyte HL-A typing. *N Engl J Med* 281:1208, 1969.

60. Herzig RH, Herzig GP, Bull MI, et al: Correction of poor platelet transfusion responses with leukocyte-poor HL-A-matched platelet concentrates. *Blood* 46:743, 1975.

61. Mittal KK, Ruder EA, Green D: Matching of histocompatibility (HL-A) antigens for platelet transfusion. *Blood* 47:31, 1976.

62. Radvany R, Green D, Rossi EC, et al: Efficacy of matched platelet transfusions from unrelated donors. *Trans Proc* IX:513, 1977.

63. Duquesnoy RJ, Filip DJ, Rodey GE, et al: Transfusion therapy of refractory thrombocytopenic patients with platelets from donors selectively mismatched for cross-reactive HLA antigens. *Trans Proc* IX:221, 1977.

64. Duquesnoy RJ, Vieira J, Aster RH: Donor availability for platelet transfusion support of alloimmunized thrombocytopenic patients. *Trans Proc* IX:519, 1977.

65. Duquesnoy RJ, Filip DJ, Rodey GE, et al: Successful transfusion of platelets "mismatched" for HLA antigens to alloimmunized thrombocytopenic patients. *Am J Hematol* 2:219, 1977.

66. Tosato G, Appelbaum FR, Deisseroth AB: HLA-matched platelet transfusion therapy of severe aplastic anemia. *Blood* 52:846, 1978.

67. Filip DJ, Duquesnoy RJ, Aster RH: Predictive value of cross-matching for transfusion of platelet concentrates to alloimmunized recipients. *Am J Hematol* 1:471, 1976.

68. Wu KK, Hoak JC, Koepke JA, et al: Selection of compatible platelet donors: a prospective evaluation of three cross-matching techniques. *Transfusion* 17:638, 1977.

69. Herzig RH, Terasaki PI, Trapani RJ, et al: The relationship between donor-recipient lymphocytotoxicity and the transfusion response using HLA-matched platelet concentrates. *Transfusion* 17:657, 1977.

70. Gmur J, von Felten A, Frick P: Platelet support in polysensitized patients: role of HLA specificities and crossmatch testing for donor selection. *Blood* 51:903, 1978.

71. Brand A, van Leeuwen A, Eernisse JG, et al: Platelet transfusion therapy. Optimal donor selection with a combination of lymphocytotoxicity and platelet fluorescence tests. *Blood* 51:781, 1978.

72. Slichter SJ: Selection of compatible platelet donors, in *Platelet Physiology and Transfusion*. Washington, DC, American Association of Blood Banks, 1978.

73. Graw RG Jr, Herzig G, Perry S, et al: Normal granulocyte transfusion therapy. *N Engl J Med* 287:367, 1972.

74. Higby DJ, Mishler JM, Cohen E, et al: Increased elevation of peripheral leukocyte counts by infusion of histocompatible granulocytes. *Vox Sang* 27:186, 1974.

75. Appelbaum FR, Trapani RJ, Graw RG Jr: Consequences of prior alloimmunization during granulocyte transfusion. *Transfusion* 17:460, 1977.

76. Westrick MA, Debelak-Fehir KM, Epstein RB: The effect of prior whole blood transfusion on subsequent granulocyte support in leukopenic dogs. *Transfusion* 17:611, 1977.

77. Ungerleider RS, Appelbaum FR, Trapani RJ, et al: Lack of predictive value of antileukocyte antibody screening in granulocyte transfusion therapy. *Transfusion* 19:90, 1979.

Chapter 4

A COMPARISON OF TECHNICS FOR LEUKAPHERESIS AND PLATELETPHERESIS

Jacob Nusbacher, MD, and James MacPherson, MS

Introduction

DURING THE PAST decade, the collection of granulocyte and platelet concentrates using automated pheresis equipment has become commonplace in both blood centers and hospital transfusion services. There has been a proliferation of machines designed for these purposes, particularly for granulocyte collection, and newer equipment is being planned or evaluated. Concomitant with these developments, there have been reported numerous modifications and technical variations of the basic technics designed to improve efficiency of collection and yields, or to enhance donor safety. Faced with this diversity, the pheresis team is sometimes at a loss as to what equipment to purchase, which approach is "best" for the needed results, and what to expect with the various methods available. The purpose of this chapter is to summarize and compare the technics available for automated pheresis, to point out some of the common technical variations and their effects on the procedure and product, and to compare the composition of the products obtained by these different methods.

Principles of Collection

Leukapheresis

Granulocytes for transfusion may be collected by two methods — centrifugation and filtration. With either technic, two venipunctures are made: one for removal of blood from the donor for processing in the collection equipment; the other, for return of blood to the donor. With the centrifugation technic, the differences in specific gravity between leukocytes and red blood cells (RBC) are exploited. This can be visualized readily by permitting a unit of whole blood to sediment; a white line, the "buffy coat" layer of leukocytes, separates the erythrocyte and plasma components. In sedimented whole blood, the buffy coat layer consists predominantly of lymphocytes, while the majority of granulocytes are still entrapped in the red cell mass. When performing centrifugation leukapheresis, a similar phenomenon occurs, making simple sampling of buffy coat an inefficient way of collecting granulocytes. Therefore, in order to improve yields of granulocytes, it is usual to use one or more of a variety of drugs that either improve RBC-granulocyte separation, or increase the donors granulocyte count. These will be discussed in greater detail below.

Filtration leukapheresis (FL) exploits the ability of granulocytes to adhere to nylon fibers in the presence of divalent cations, such as calcium. Only heparin may be used as an anticoagulant because of this latter requirement. Blood is propelled through a pair of nylon-filled plastic tubes (Leukopak™* filters) in a continuous-flow manner. The granulocytes adhere to the nylon, while other blood elements return to the donor. After the collection procedure is terminated, granulocytes are retrieved from the nylon packs by perfusion with a calcium-chelating citrate solution.

Plateletpheresis

Viable platelets may be separated from whole blood only by centrifugation. Platelets have a specific gravity significantly different from red cells or granulocytes, but more like lymphocytes. The centrifugation methods used for platelet harvesting are similar to those used for granulocyte collection, but pharmacological additives are not necessary. However, platelet concentrates will contain large numbers of lymphocytes (and some red blood cells) unless these are removed specifically after the plateletpheresis procedure.

Equipment

Table 1 presents an overview of the equipment currently available for performing pheresis. With the exception of filtration leukapheresis, all equipment is multipurpose. In practice, however, it is unusual to find a pheresis unit fully operational with only one machine. Demands for granulocyte or platelet concentrates (as well as for therapeutic procedures) are often episodic and frequently require performing a number of procedures daily, and perhaps simultaneously. Therefore, a self-sufficient pheresis program requires more than one machine and perhaps different kinds of machines. The decision as to which format to acquire can be made only after an analysis of the specific requirements of the program and the relative availability of funds.

---

* TM-Fenwal Laboratories, Deerfield, Ill.

Aminco or IBM/NCI Cell Separator

The first machine for granulocyte collection was developed at the National Cancer Institute in collaboration with the IBM Corporation. It is now marketed only by American Instruments Corporation. This cell separator operates on a continuous-flow principle. Blood is pumped into a centrifuge bowl where separation of red cell, buffy coat, and plasma layers is accomplished. Specially designed sampling ports on the top of the bowl remove each of these three blood elements separately. The red cells and plasma are recombined and returned to the donor; the buffy coat is collected in a bag. An important feature of this machine, par-

Table 1. — Some Fundamental Aspects of Cytopheresis Collection Equipment

	Aminco¶	Haemonetics Model 30	IBM 2997	Filtration (Fenwal)
Capital Cost*	$19,000	$18,800	$25,900	$2,700
Software Cost**	$110	$70	$70	$70
Collection Apparatus	reusable	expendable	expendable	expendable
Type of collection				
granulocytes	+	+	+	+
platelets	±***	+	+	−
Therapeutics	+	+	+	−
Type of Flow	continuous	intermittent	continuous	continuous
Ex vivo volume (ml)	<250	425-500□	<200	<250
Anticoagulation	citrate	citrate	citrate	heparin

  * Approximate.
  ** Varies with technic and type of collection.
  *** Not usually used. Data in literature are sparse.
  ¶ Smaller machine with disposable bowl in late developmental stage.
  □ Varies with Hct. 600 ml more with 375 ml bowl.
Note: Does not include new Fenwal CS 3000 which is currently being evaluated for leukapheresis and plateletpheresis.

ticularly when performing therapeutic pheresis on anemic donors, is the low ex vivo blood volume of about 250 ml.

The machine requires full-time operator attention in order to adjust the location of buffy coat layer at the site of the white cell collection ports. This is accomplished by adjusting the flow rate of RBC relative to plasma exiting from the bowl. Blood flow rates depend on the patency of the donor's veins and the dwell time in the bowl that is required for effective separation of the blood components. For these reasons, it is unusual to be able to achieve flow rates of more than 60 ml per minute in normal donors and get component separation. This machine is somewhat complex to set up and cannot be moved readily. The centrifuge bowl is reusable and requires sterilization (a reusable bowl is being developed). The bowl tends to develop cracks after about 50 autoclavings.

Production of this machine is being phased out, to be replaced by a smaller one with disposable software and employing a nonrotating seal.[1]

Haemonetics Model 30

This centrifuge operates on an intermittent-flow principle. Blood is pumped into a centrifuge bowl where separation of the blood components occurs. The plasma, being the lightest constituent, exits from the bowl first and is collected in a bag. The next layers are the platelet and/or leukocyte layers (depending on which blood element is desired, or both) which exit from the bowl next and are collected in a second bag. The centrifuge is then stopped; the red blood cells remaining in the bowl and the supernatant plasma that was initially collected are pumped into a bag for reinfusion, by gravity, into the donor's other arm. While the reinfusion is occurring, a second "pass" through the bowl may be initiated. In the usual procedure, six "passes" through the large bowl (375 ml), or eight "passes" through the small bowl (225 ml) are done. It is unusual to perform more extensive pheresis (more passes) for the collection of either granulocytes or platelets because, with either type of cell collection, large numbers of platelets are collected, resulting in a significant fall in the donor's platelet count (see below). The ex vivo volume with this machine is relatively large: a minimum of 750 ml with the large bowl and 450 ml with the small bowl, assuming a donor hematocrit of 40%. In practice, there is little time saved in using the large bowl and there is some evidence that for platelet collection, the smaller bowl is slightly more efficient.[2]

IBM 2997

This continuous-flow centrifuge has become available recently. Its format and general characteristics are similar to the older IBM-Aminco equipment. The centrifuge bowl has been replaced by disposable hoop-like separation modules. There are two such modules, one for granulocyte collection; the other, for plateletpheresis. As compared with the older formats, this machine is more fully automated, particularly with regard to the proper placement of the buffy coat interface at the proper sampling port. The ex vivo volume with this machine is less than 170 ml.

Filtration Leukapheresis

This technic may be used only for granulocyte collection. The hardware consists of only a simple roller pump. All software is disposable.

Donor blood flow rates with the technic depend only on the capacity of the donor's veins and may reach 100 ml per minute, although 60 ml per minute is more usual. The ex vivo volume is small (240 ml). As granulocytes are the only blood cells that are removed significantly, and these are immediately replaced into the circulation from tissue stores, the procedure may, in theory, proceed for a long time for greater collection yields. Unfortunately, the loading capacity of the two parallel filters may limit yields to a maximum of about 3×10^{10} granulocytes[3,4] which, in the usual donor, occurs after about 8-10 liters of donor blood have been processed. Thus, there is little point in continuing the procedure beyond this point unless a fresh set of filters is used. The latter technic has been reported to be useful in achieving higher yields.[5] Using four filters in parallel also achieves higher yields.[6]

To retrieve the granulocytes that have adhered to the nylon, the filters must be eluted with a calcium-chelating solution.[3] The usual approach is to pass through the filters about 1000 ml of a solution consisting of 250 ml of ACD (or an equivalent concentrated sodium citrate solution), 200-400 ml CPD plasma and made up to 1000 ml with saline. Gentle tapping of the filters with a blunt instrument helps free the cells from the nylon. The eluted material is then centrifuged at $250 \times g$ for 15 minutes at 4 C to concentrate the cells in a volume of less than 250 ml.

Pharmacologic Manipulation to Increase Yields

While there are no good data on how many granulocytes constitute a therapeutic "dose" for granulocyte transfusion, it generally is assumed that the larger the dose, the better. As a rule of thumb, many blood centers strive to collect at least 1×10^{10} granulocytes per procedure. With centrifugation leukapheresis, because of the similarity in specific gravity between granulocytes and red blood cells, and because of the paucity of granulocytes relative to RBC in the circulation, it is difficult — impossible — to achieve this yield in collected cells unless the duration of the leukapheresis procedure is prolonged unduly. Two strategies have been developed to improve the efficiency, and thus the yield, in leukapheresis procedures. The first approach is to increase the donor's granulocyte count by the administration of certain steroid drugs; the second is to improve the separation of RBC and granulocytes in the separation module through the use of RBC sedimenting agents.

Administration of adrenocorticosteroids has been known to produce a granulocytosis since the introduction of this class of drugs in the 1950s.[7] In leukapheresis programs, it has been demonstrated that pretreatment of donors with prednisone,[8] dexamethasone[9] or other steroid drugs[10,11] increases the donor's prepheresis granulocyte count by 50% to 100% and results in a commensurate increase in the number of functionally normal granulocytes collected. To achieve maximal benefit, it is critical to time the administration of these drugs so that the peak granulocytosis is achieved prior to the pheresis procedure.[12] Table 2 lists some of the steroid drugs now in use, routes of administration, dosages, and time to achieve peak effects. Corticosteroid pretreatment is efficacious in both centrifugation[8-11] and filtration leukapheresis.[8,13]

A second, independent approach to increasing yields is by the use of RBC sedimenting agents. This is applicable only to centrifugation leukapheresis and requires the introduction of RBC rouleaux-inducing agents into the blood as it leaves the donor's arm. Improved RBC-granulocyte separation occurs in the separation equipment resulting in an approximate doubling of yields. Two drugs have been used for this purpose — dextran[14] and hydroxyethyl starch (HES)[15] — although, in the United

Table 2. — Corticosteroid pretreatment to Increase Granulocyte Yields in Leukapheresis

Drug	Dose/Route of Administration	Time Prior to Pheresis (Hrs)
Prednisone	60 mg p.o.	4-12
Dexamethasone	6-8 mg i.v.	4-6
Dexamethasone	6-8 mg/m² p.o.	4-6
Dexamethasone/double dose	3 mg/m² p.o.	12
	3 mg/m² p.o.	3
Hydrocortisone	120 mg/m² i.v.	2.5-6

States, HES seems to be preferred, perhaps because of its somewhat lower immunogenicity as compared with dextran. Usually, HES is administered as a 6% solution delivered at a ratio of 1 ml for every 8-12 ml of donor blood. The effects of steroids and HES, when used in combination, are additive.[16]

Yields

Plateletpheresis

Most automated plateletpheresis procedures are done with the Haemonetics Model 30 apparatus. The recently-introduced IBM 2997 apparatus has a specific platelet collection module, but there are, as yet, little data on the machine's efficacy in this regard. An even newer apparatus, developed by Fenwal, is still in the evaluation stage.

The typical yields of all blood elements obtained with the Haemonetics Model 30 are shown in Table 3. Large numbers of platelets are harvested after six passes on the large bowl or eight passes with the small bowl (mean volume of blood processed of approximately 4 liters). About 56% of all platelets processed are recovered in the final product (see reference 2 for detail of this calculation).

Platelet concentrates obtained with this equipment are contaminated significantly with lymphocytes and red blood cells (the equivalent of 50 ml whole blood for the latter). Considerations of erythrocyte and/or leukocyte compatibility may make necessary the removal of these cells prior to transfusion. This can be accomplished readily by an additional centrifugation of the final product at $150 \times g$ for 7 minutes at 22 C, and careful removal of the supernatant for transfusion. This procedure can result in the removal of 92% and more than 99% of the contaminating lymphocytes and red cells respectively, but with a loss of nearly 20%

Table 3. — Typical Yields After Plateletpheresis with the Haemonetics Model 30 Blood Cell Processor*

Platelets — 5.5×10^{11}
Lymphocytes — $1.8–4.1 \times 10^{9}$
Other leukocytes — $1-4 \times 10^{8}$
Hemoglobin — 5 gm
Volume — 250 ml

* 4 liters processed, compiled from Ref. 2.

---

of the harvested platelets.[2] Despite this, we perform the added centrifugation routinely, because there is some evidence that lymphocyte contamination of platelet concentrates may be an important factor in reducing efficacy of platelet transfusion in the alloimmunized recipient.[17] The IBM 2997 apparatus has been reported to yield about 4.5×10^{11} platelets per procedure, with an efficiency comparable to the Haemonetics machine.

Yields in plateletpheresis procedures are directly proportional to the donor's prepheresis platelet count.[18] Thus, preselection of donors on this basis, if possible, would increase yields substantially. Unfortunately, increased yields cannot be readily obtained by processing more donor blood, that is, increasing the number of passes through the separation bowl. In the usual procedure, the donor's platelet count falls by approximately one-third. Increased processing would thus increase the risk of postpheresis donor thrombocytopenia. In almost all cases, the usual yields obtained are more than adequate as a therapeutic dose.

Leukapheresis

Aminco Celltrifuge I/IBM-NCI Blood Cell Processor. Table 4 summarizes the typical yields obtained with this format of leukapheresis equipment. The data are collated from a number of different publications and should be considered approximations. Variations in technical details may affect yields somewhat.

As with all centrifugation methods, yields of granulocytes using this equipment without any pharmacologic manipulation are poor. The use of HES and/or corticosteroid pretreatment is believed to be a necessity by most investigators. The granulocytes collected with this equipment have normal function.[19,20] This machine — the first leukapheresis equipment to be developed — has been the mainstay of a number of active pheresis units throughout the country and, with proper operator training, performs

Table 4. — Typical Yields After Leukapheresis with the Aminco Celltrifuge I/IBM-NCL Blood Cell Processors*

Granulocytes	
No Additives	0.6×10^{10}
HES	1.0×10^{10}
Steroids	1.0×10^{10}
Steroids & HES	2.0×10^{10}
Other Leukocytes	0.7×10^{10}
Platelets	$20\text{-}70 \times 10^{10}$
Hemoglobin	9 g
Volume	300-500 ml

* Values are for 9 liters processed per procedure (3 hours).
Compiled from Refs. 8, 11, 15, 16, 21, 32-34.

efficiently and consistently, particularly for granulocyte collection. In the literature, there are much less data on its value as a platelet harvesting apparatus.[21] It is also highly effective for therapeutic cytopheresis and plasma exchanges.

Haemonetics Model 30 Blood Cell Processor. Table 5 summarizes typical yields obtained with this equipment. Here again, the need for pharmacologic manipulation is mandatory; we are not aware of any pheresis unit that is using the Haemonetics Model 30 without HES. One important advantage of this equipment is the large number of platelets obtained as a "contaminant." As many recipients of granulocytes are also thrombocytopenic, this feature is especially attractive. Alternatively, the granulocytes and platelets can be separated from each other for transfusions into two different recipients. This is accomplished by centrifugation at $70 \times g$ for seven minutes at 22 C, with removal of the platelet-rich supernatant.

56

The Haemonetics Model 30 has achieved rather wide acceptance in the blood bank community because of its versatility, relative ease of use, and portability. It has been used frequently for therapeutic cytopheresis and plasma exchange, although it is perhaps somewhat less desirable than other formats for some patients, because of the high ex vivo volume.

Filtration Leukapheresis. Table 6 summarizes the typical yields obtained with this technic. This method of leukapheresis results in the large

Table 5. — Typical Yields After Leukapheresis with the Haemonetics Model 30 Blood Cell Processor*

Granulocytes	
No Additives	**
HES	1.3×10^{10}
HES + Steroids	1.9×10^{10}
Other Leukocytes	0.4×10^{10}
Platelets	60×10^{10}
Hemoglobin	9 g
Volume	300-500 ml

* Values are for 4 liters processed per procedure (2½ hrs).
** <10% collection efficiency.
Compiled from Refs. 35-37.

Table 6. — Typical Yields After Leukapheresis by Filtration Leukapheresis*

Granulocytes	
Unstimulated	2.0×10^{10}
Steroids	2.8×10^{10}
4 Filters (Parallel)	3.6×10^{10}
Other Leukocytes	$<0.1 \times 10^{10}$
Platelets**	1.25×10^{11}
Hemoglobin	6 g
Volume	150-350 ml

* Yields for average 2-2½ hour procedures.
** Platelets have reduced in vivo survival.
Compiled from Refs. 8, 38, 39.

number of granulocytes collected and with a relatively small number of other contaminating cells. Conceptually, this is the ideal technic for granulocyte harvesting, but, unfortunately, a variety of associated problems have severely restricted its use throughout the United States. These can be summarized as follows: possible hazards to the donor, including the mandatory requirement for heparin anticoagulation; the occurrence of perineal (abdominal) pain in some (usually female) donors (reported mitigated by corticosteroid pretreatment);[22] the demonstration of complement activation during this procedure;[23] and two reports of donor priapism. Furthermore, the quality of cells obtained by filtration leukapheresis has been found defective by some investigators[20,24-26] (but not by others),[27-29] and there is a high incidence of recipient reactions when compared with other methods.[30,31] (This latter effect may result from the use of excessive centrifugation rates when concentrating the final product prior to transfusion. Centrifugation at $250 \times g$ is recommended.) Despite these considerations, it is clear that granulocytes obtained by FL are effective in the treatment of septic neutropenic patients and laboratory animals.

IBM 2997. Table 7 summarizes leukapheresis yields obtained with this apparatus. This equipment has been introduced only recently; published data are sparse and are available only in abstract form. The use of HES with this apparatus appears to be necessary.

Table 7. — Typical Yields After Leukapheresis with the IBM 2997 Blood Cell Processor*

Granulocytes	
No Additives	No data
HES	1.1×10^{10}
Steroids	No data
Steroids & HES	2.6×10^{10}
Other Leukocytes	$.7-.9 \times 10^{10}$
Platelets	No data

* From Ref. 40.

References

1. Ito Y, Suaudeau J, Bowman RL: New flow-through centrifuge without rotating seals applied to plasmapheresis. *Science* 189:999, 1975.
2. Nusbacher J, Sher ML, MacPherson JL: Plateletpheresis using the Haemonetics Model 30 cell separator. *Vox Sang* 33:9, 1977.
3. Herzig GP, Root RK, Graw RG: Granulocyte collection by continuous-flow filtration leukapheresis. *Blood* 39:554, 1972.
4. MacPherson JL, Wiltbank TB, Yagnow RL, et al: Studies of granulocyte adhesion during filtration leukapheresis and in vitro, abstracted. *Transfusion* 18:651, 1978.
5. Djerassi I, Kim JS, Suvansri U, et al: Filtration leukapheresis: Principles and techniques for harvesting and transfusion of filtered granulocytes and monocytes, Golman JM, Lowenthal RM (eds): in

Leucocytes: Separation, Collection and Transfusion. Academic Press, London, 1975, pp 123-136.

6. Hill NO, Khan A, Hill JM, et al: Granulocyte preparation by continuous-flow filtration leukapheresis, in *Leukocytes: Separation, Collection and Transfusion,* op. cit. pp 168-173.

7. Athens JW, Haab OP, Raab SO, et al: The mechanism of steroid granulocytosis. *J Clin Invest* 41:1342, 1962.

8. MacPherson JL, Nusbacher J, Bennett JM: The acquisition of granulocytes by leukapheresis: A comparison of continuous-flow centrifugation and filtration leukapheresis in normal and corticosteroid-stimulated donors. *Transfusion* 16:221, 1976.

9. Higby DJ, Mishler JM, Rhomberg W, et al: The effect of a single or double dose of dexamethasone on granulocyte collection with the continuous flow centrifuge. *Vox Sang* 28:243, 1975.

10. Shoji M, Vogler RW: Effects of hydrocortisone on yield and bactericidal function of granulocytes collected by continuous-flow centrifugation. *Blood* 44:435, 1974.

11. McCredie KB, Freireich EJ: The use of etiocholanolone to increase collection of granulocytes with the IBM blood cell separator. *J Clin Invest* 49:63a, 1970.

12. Mishler JM: The effects of corticosteroids on mobilization and function of neutrophils. *Exp Hematol* 5 (sup):15, 1977.

13. Higby DJ, Henderson ES, Burnett D, et al: Filtration leukapheresis: Effects of donor stimulation with dexamethasone. *Blood* 50:953, 1977.

14. Lowenthal RM, Park DS: The use of dextran as an adjunct to granulocyte collection on the continuous-flow blood cell separator. *Transfusion* 15:23, 1975.

15. Mishler JM, Hadlock DE, Fortuny IE, et al: Increased efficiency of leukocyte separation by addition of hydroxyethyl starch to the continuous-flow centrifuge. *Blood* 44:571, 1974.

16. Mishler JM, Higby DJ, Rhomberg W: Hydroxyethyl starch, and dexamethasone as an adjunct to leukocyte separation with the IBM blood cell separator. *Transfusion* 14:352, 1974.

17. Herzig RH, Herzig GP, Bull MI, et al: Correction of poor platelet responses with leukocyte-poor HLA-matched platelet concentrates. *Blood* 46:743, 1975.

18. Szymanski IO, Patti K, Kliman A: Efficacy of the Latham blood processor to perform plateletpheresis. *Transfusion* 13:405, 1973.

19. Graw RG Jr, Herzig GP, Perry S, et al: Normal granulocyte transfusion therapy. Treatment of septicemia due to gram-negative bacteria. *N Engl J Med* 287:367, 1972.

20. McCullough J, Weiblen BJ, Deinard, et al: In vitro function and post-transfusion survival of granulocytes collected by continuous-flow centrifugation and by filtration leukapheresis. *Blood* 48:315, 1976.

21. Graw RG Jr, Herzig GP, Eisel RJ, et al: Leukocyte and platelet collection from normal donors with the continuous-flow blood cell separator. *Transfusion* 11:94, 1971.

22. Wiltbank TB, Nusbacher J, Higby DJ, et al: Abdominal pain in donors during filtration leukapheresis. *Transfusion* 17:159, 1977.

23. Nusbacher J, Rosenfeld SI, MacPherson JL, et al: Nylon fiber leukapheresis: Associated complement component changes and granulocytopenia. *Blood* 51:359, 1978.

24. Roy AJ, Yankee RA, Brivkalns A, et al: Viability of granulocytes collected by filtration leukapheresis. *Transfusion* 15:539, 1975.

25. Wright DG, Kauffman JC, Chusid MJ, et al: Functional abnormalities of human neutrophils collected by continuous-flow filtration leukapheresis. *Blood* 46:901, 1975.

26. Applebaum FR, Norton L, Graw RG Jr: Migration of transfused granulocytes in leukopenic dogs. *Blood* 49:483, 1977.

27. Harris MB, Djerassi I, Schwartz E, et al: Polymorphonuclear leukocytes prepared by continuous-flow filtration leukapheresis. Viability and Function. *Blood* 44:707, 1974.

28. Steigbigel RT, Baum J, MacPherson JL, et al: Granulocyte bactericidal capacity and chemotaxis as affected by continuous-flow centrifugation and filtration leukapheresis, steroid administration and storage. *Blood* 53:197, 1978.

29. Alavi JB, Root RK, Djerassi I, et al: A randomized clinical trial of granulocyte transfusion for infection in acute leukemia. *N Engl J Med* 296:706, 1977.

30. Higby DJ, Henderson ES, Holland JF: Filtration leukapheresis for granulocyte transfusion therapy. *N Engl J Med* 292:15, 1975.

31. Schiffer CA, Buchholz D, Aisner J, et al: Clinical experience with transfusion of granulocytes obtained by continuous-flow filtration leukapheresis. *Am J Med* 58:373, 1975.

32. Clift RA, Buckner CD, Williams BM, et al: Improved granulocyte procurement with the continuous flow centrifuge. *Transfusion* 13:276, 1973.

33. Koza I, Holland JF, Cohen E. Histocompatible leukocyte transfusions during granulocytopenia. *Neoplasma* 18:185, 1971.

34. McCredie KB, Freireich EJ, Hester JP, et al: Increased granulocyte collection using the blood cell separator and the addition of etiocholanolone and hydroxyethyl starch. *Transfusion* 14:357, 1974.

35. Aisner J, Schiffer CA, Wolff JH, et al: A standardized technique for efficient platelet and leukocyte collection using the Model 30 blood processor. *Transfusion* 16:437, 1976.
36. Huestis DW, Goodsite LM, Price MJ, et al: Granulocyte collection with the Haemonetics blood cell processor, in *Leucocytes: Separation, collection and transfusion,* op. cit, pp 208-218.
37. Patten E, Young A, Mercer C. The combined use of granulocytes and platelet transfusions using the Haemonetics Model 30 blood processor, in *Proceedings of the Haemonetics Research Institute Advanced Component Seminar.* Boston, 1978.
38. Djerassi I, Kim JS, Suvansri U, et al: Continuous-flow filtration-leukapheresis. *Transfusion* 12:75, 1972.
39. Kernoff L, Schackleton D, Dubovsky D, et al: Studies on platelets contained in eluates following filtration leukapheresis. *Transfusion* 19:114, 1979.
40. Hester JP, Kellogg RM, Mulzet A, et al: Component collection and transfusion: The IBM 2997 disposable system, abstracted, in *Proceedings Third International Leukocyte Conference on Collection and Transfusion.* Chicago, 1978.

Chapter 5

PHERESIS DONOR REACTIONS AND COMPLICATIONS: PREVENTION, RECOGNITION AND MANAGEMENT

Letty Kotwas, BS, RN

Introduction

THE GREAT DEMAND for blood components has led to many technological advances. Since the development of pheresis for the collection of transfusable platelets and leukocytes, we have advanced from an era of pioneers to the establishment of cytopheresis as a routine service. With the rapid development of pheresis centers, it is worth emphasizing the risks, side effects, and complications of pheresis procedures on normal healthy donors. It is necessary to understand the potential adverse effects on donors and to plan for their prevention, recognition and management prior to the institution of a pheresis program. Prevention and early recognition have great importance in ensuring both a safe procedure for the donor and a quality product for the recipient. The purpose of this chapter is to discuss the recognition and management of these side effects and complications that may develop in pheresis donors.

Donor Preparation

The physical and emotional status of the pheresis donor is important in ensuring a successful pheresis procedure. Anxiety is a predisposing factor leading to syncopal reactions.[1] A pheresis donor who has been a regular whole blood donor possesses a comfortable perception of his/her donation capabilities and health status. In contrast, anxiety may flood the family member whose first intense experience is a pheresis procedure which often requires frequent donations. Many respond to this challenge excellently. Some become irritable and demanding. Others try to flee by not showing for appointments. Many, however, appreciate the opportunity to talk about the critical nature of this family problem. All pheresis donors, whether they be nonrelated volunteers or family members, require the support of an understanding and professional staff. A sensitivity to the donor's attitude is essential.

Anxiety is reduced by a thorough explanation of the procedures and the equipment involved. A brief explanation of the recipient's blood needs substantiates the importance of the donation. Disorganization on the part of the pheresis staff undermines confidence. Confidence in the personnel is key to a successful program. A thorough medical history screening, a careful choice of venipuncture sites, and the start of the procedure in an efficient manner, without delay, can be very reassuring. Venipuncture delays and manipulations of the needle may result in anxiety and precipitate vagal reactions, even in seasoned donors. Intradermal 1% lidocaine can be used, resulting in a painless venipuncture for selected donors.

General Complications or Risks of Donating Blood

Venipuncture site infection or inflammation may occur despite a thorough, careful venipuncture preparation technic. The development of redness, swelling, and tenderness 24 hours or more following a procedure should prompt an assessment by the pheresis physician. Postdonation bleeding from the venipuncture site should be treated with elevation and direct pressure with a dry sterile dressing.

Iron Depletion

Any blood donation containing red cells carries with it the risk of donor iron depletion at a rate of 1 mg per ml of red cells withdrawn. The risk of iron depletion depends upon the hematocrit of the pheresis product and the frequency of donation. Depending upon technic, the hematocrit may vary between zero and 30%. Each center should be aware of red cell quantity of the pheresis product and the number of donor samples removed (routine processing, quality control, crossmatching, HLA typing, research). The maximum number of pheresis donations per eight-week period can be determined so that no more than 250 mg of iron (equivalent to one unit of whole blood) is withdrawn each eight weeks.

Complications and Risks Related to Pheresis

A variety of risks and side effects accompany pheresis procedures. These result from various causes and may be grouped generally into degrees of severity: mild, moderate, and severe. Mild symptoms not given early attention may progress to a moderate or severe degree. Mild reactions are alterations in the donor's status that are easily corrected. Some mild reactions include the following: restlessness, yawning, sighing, mild perspiration, pallor, hyperventilation, tachycardia, nausea, sneezing, chills, dizziness, lightheadedness, nasal stuffiness, scleral redness, transient perineal, perianal or scrotal burning, and mild citrate-induced parethesias.

Moderate reactions require more intervention and must be reversed before the procedure can continue. A moderate reaction can be a progression of a mild reaction. Loss of consciousness preceded by bradycardia and hypotension, or striking citrate reactions, are examples. Treatment is the same as for mild reactions.

Severe reactions result in termination of the procedure and may be displayed as tetanic contractions of the extremities, marked shortness of breath, chest heaviness or pain, prolonged hypovolemic or vagal hypotensive reactions with convulsions or cyanosis, allergic reactions, the abdominal pain syndrome or menorrhagia. Technical failures or complications of the procedure, such as hemolysis or air embolism, may lead to severe reaction and immediate termination of the procedure.

Mild Syncopal or Vasovagal Reactions

Vasovagal or syncopal reactions usually are gradual in onset and often can be reversed readily when recognized in the early stages. These reactions occur no more frequently during pheresis donations than during whole blood donations.[2] Vasovagal reactions may be described as mild when consisting of restlessness, pallor, lightheadedness, diaphoresis, or hyperventilation. Mild reactions are readily reversed by:

1. Diverting the donor's attention with conversation.
2. Slowing or temporarily discontinuing the extraction of blood.
3. Tilting the donation chair, lowering the head, and elevating the feet slightly.
4. Infusing saline.

Prevention of syncopal reactions should be the goal:

1. Reduce donor apprehension and anxiety.
2. Reinfuse platelet-poor or leukocyte-poor blood at a rate equal to or greater than the withdrawal rate.
3. Select the pheresis bowl size that corresponds to the donor's weight or body surface area.

Severe Vasovagal and Hypovolemic Reactions

The risk of hypotension and syncope is great when the amount of blood removed in the recumbent position approaches or exceeds 15% to 20% (800-1200 ml) of the donor's total blood volume.[3] The effect of blood loss on the cardiovascular response can be detected by changing the donor's position from supine to sitting. The degree of pulse and blood pressure change reflects the amount of blood removed acutely (Table 1). This is particularly important in the small donors whose extracorporeal volume to total blood volume ratio may be relatively great. It often is wise to infuse isotonic saline as the first portion of blood is removed from small donors.

During filtration leukapheresis (FL) and continuous-flow centrifugation (CFC), the total extracorporeal volume is approximately 250 ml. Using the Haemonetics Model 30, the extracorporeal volume is dependent upon the bowl size selected and the donor's hematocrit (Table 2).

Severe reactions with prolonged loss of consciousness, convulsions, tetany, carpalpedal spasms or cyanosis are treated as follows:

1. Discontinue the procedure.
2. Maintain intravenous patency with isotonic saline.
3. Notify the pheresis physician.
4. Tilt the donor chair to lower head and elevate feet.

Table 1.— Cardiovascular Response to Position Change Depends Upon Volume of Blood Removed

Blood Volume Removed (ml)	Supine		Sitting	
	Blood Pressure	Pulse	Blood Pressure	Pulse
none	normal	normal	normal	normal
500	normal	normal	normal	N or ↑
1000	normal	N or ↑	N or ↓	↑
1500	N or ↓	↑	↓	↑ or ↓
2000	↓	↑ or ↓	↓↓	↑ or ↓

Data from: Candon RE, **Manual Surg Therapeutics,** 1969.

Table 2. — Volume of Blood in Extracorporeal Circuit Using Haemonetics Model 30 Blood Processor Depends upon Donor Hematocrit and Bowl Size

Hematocrit	Extracorporeal Volume (ml)	
	225 ml Bowl	375 ml Bowl
38%	473	789
41%	439	731
45%	400	666
48%	375	625

Hyperventilation

Hyperventilation is often the result of an underlying anxiety. Symptoms such as blurring of vision, breathlessness, numbness, and tingling are common symptoms. Symptoms of hyperventilation resulting from the loss of carbon dioxide, leading to a shift of blood pH and hypocal-

cemia due to increased binding by albumin, may be ameliorated by having
the donor breathe into a paper bag. Early signs, such as deep sighing,
which may accompany restlessness, should be noted even before symptoms develop. Mild hyperventilation may accompany and complicate
syncopal reactions. Intervention may require diverting the donor's attention, slowing the extraction, infusing saline, or tilting the chair.

Transient Perineal, Perianal, or Scrotal Burning or Tingling Sensations

Transient perineal, perianal, or scrotal burning or tingling sensations
have been observed briefly at the onset of leukapheresis immediately following administration of intravenous heparin and dexamethasone. Ordinarily, this is transient, infrequent, and requires no immediate treatment.
It is best prevented by slow injection of intravenous medicines over
a three- to four-minute period.

Scleral Redness

Scleral redness has been observed transiently during the initial portion
of FL. At times, it is accompanied by a facial flushing, nasal stuffiness,
sneezing, and a watery "glassy-eyed" appearance. It is not known whether
this is caused by the intravenous medications or by the initial interaction
of blood with nylon filters. It is self-limited and requires no specific
therapy.

Heparin

Heparin may produce donor complications because of bleeding or
allergic reactions. Bleeding complications due to heparin ordinarily are
not serious and usually have been limited to postpheresis bleeding at the
venipuncture site. Menorrhagia is rare. The length of time heparin
remains active in the circulation depends upon individual sensitivity and
the dose administered. Treatment of persistent postpheresis venipuncture
bleeding following FL may include application of pressure dressings and
elevation; if venipuncture bleeding persists longer than 30 minutes, the
pheresis physician should be consulted to determine whether protamine
should be given to neutralize the heparin action.

Hemorrhagic complications due to heparin are largely prevented by
avoiding use in donors with:

1. Current menstruation.
2. Active peptic ulcer disease or gastrointestinal bleeding within the
   past 2 years.
3. Hypertension.

4. History of bleeding tendency.
5. History of chronic aspirin use.

If bleeding develops after the donor has left the blood center, have the donor return immediately or go to the nearest hospital emergency room for evaluation.

Protamine Sulfate

Protamine Sulfate is used by a few pheresis centers to neutralize the effects of heparin. The risks of using protamine are centered around its cardiac and allergic effects. The drug must be administered slowly at less than 10 mg per minute in order to avoid symptoms of flushing, dyspnea, tachycardia, and hypotension. Donors with an allergy to fish may be hypersensitive to protamine.[4] Treatment of allergic reactions is discussed below.

Hydroxyethyl Starch

Hydroxyethyl Starch (HES) is a red cell sedimenting agent used during centrifugation leukapheresis in order to increase neutrophil yields. HES has been used successfully in thousands of procedures;[5] however, its long-term effects are unknown.

HES is metabolized into smaller molecules which are excreted in urine and feces. When a donor is given 500 ml of 6% HES, 39% is excreted in the urine during the first 24 hours. Because of the persistence of 57%-65% of the administered dose, HES given daily can have a cumulative and volume-expansion effect for 24 hours or more.[6,7] Although progressively eliminated from the tissues, animal models have retained very low levels of HES for several months.[5]

After more than a million high doses, no fatal anaphylactoid reactions have been reported. In one study, 8 of 10,273 patients exhibited anaphylactoid reactions including 3 with rashes, 3 with tachycardia, and 2 with mild hypotension. In another report, involving 16,405 large doses, the incidence of mild rashes was 0.03% nausea, tachycardia, hypotension, or respiratory disturbance was 0.05%, and marked hypotension was 0.006%.[8]

In summary, HES is stored transiently in tissues, predominantly in phagocytic cells, and is metabolized and eliminated from the body. However, the long-term effects of HES are unknown.

HES, when used in doses common for leukapheresis, does not carry with it a risk of bleeding. The platelet function, prothrombin time, partial thromboplastin time, and bleeding time are unchanged, **even when** used with the usual citrate.[5,9]

Donors have experienced temporary weight gain, headache, and pyrogenic reactions infrequently. These are self-limited and require only symptomatic treatment. Because of the volume expansion effect of HES, it is best to avoid using it in donors with hypertension, even if controlled, or with donors who tend to develop leg edema.

Hypersensitivity and Allergic Reactions

Allergic reactions may be observed in pheresis donors due to administered medications. For acute urticaria:

1. Stop procedure.
2. Maintain intravenous patency with isotonic saline.
3. Notify pheresis physician.
4. Give diphenhydromine 50 mg orally or intramuscularly.

For urticaria accompanied by hypotension, faintness, oropharyngeal edema (anaphylactoid reaction):

1. Stop procedure.
2. Maintain intravenous patency with isotonic saline.
3. Notify pheresis physician.
4. Give epinephrine 0.3 ml SC, diphenhydramine 50 mg IM or IV and dexamethasone 6 mg IM or IV.

Corticosteroid Premedication

Corticosteroid premedication frequently is given to raise the neutrophil count and improve yields. After a single dose, a few donors may experience insomnia, excitability, anxiety, increased sense of well-being or talkativeness. These occasional side effects of a single dose are self-limited and usually require only reassurance. Daily use may cause weight gain, hyperglycemia, hypertension, and mood alterations. With the usual doses given for leukapheresis, the frequency of steroid administration should be limited to no more than twice per week.

Chilliness

Chilliness may develop in the pheresis donor, varying from a mild coolness of the hands and feet, to true shaking chills (rigors). This side effect may be associated with any type of pheresis and may be attributable to immobilization in an air-conditioned environment and to the cooling of the blood during extracorporeal circulation. However, there appears no consistent change in body temperature. Countermeasures include:

1. Prevention by keeping the environment comfortably warm.
2. Blankets.
3. Warm fluids.

Paresthesias

The reinfusion of citrated blood and the accompanying transient hypocalcemia are thought to be responsible for various paresthesias during pheresis. The rapid rate of citrate reinfusion, exceeding the rate with which it is metabolized, provides a basis for the hypocalcemic symptoms experienced. Paresthesias are the more frequent donor side effects experienced during plateletpheresis. Frequently, paresthesias are described as circumoral or facial numbness or tingling, coolness of the throat, or a feeling as though the donor chair were vibrating from contact with the blood processor. The trunk may become affected upon subsequent returns of citrated blood. Donors may notice they feel cold and begin to shiver. Their muscles may begin to twitch. A general feeling of nervousness may be present with nausea or vomiting being unusual.

Although these symptoms often are associated with the return of citrated blood, they may occur at any time. The first sign to the donor usually is the circumoral effect. Instruct the donor to mention any numbness or tingling. This is an indication to slow the flow rate of the returning citrated blood. Symptoms should subside in two to three minutes. During intermittent-flow plateletpheresis (Haemonetics), citrated whole blood is returned at a rate of 500 ml every 10 to 20 minutes. In a 70 kg male, using ACD-A, this would be an equivalent infusion rate of 1.2-3.0 mg/kg/min. Using ACD-B, this would be an equivalent infusion rate of 0.74 to 1.85 mg/kg/min.

Citrate-induced paresthesias occur frequently and seem harmless, but still represent a serious risk to the pheresis donor. There is a transient lowering of the serum calcium and electrocardiographic changes with the cyclic reinfusion of citrated blood during plateletpheresis.[10-13] In a study of 15 procedures using ACD-A (3% citrate) the rate of citrate reinfusion was 1.2-2.1 mg/kg/min. Citrate loads of this magnitude were not associated with cardiac problems or hypotension, but all donors who received citrate at a rate of greater than 1.5 mg/kg/min experienced symptoms.[11] These effects of citrate are very transient due to rapid metabolism of citrate by the liver, perhaps because of redistribution of citrate into the extracellular space and release of calcium from the bone. Administration of IV calcium is an unnecessary treatment for normal donors.

Others have demonstrated that citrate infusion rates of 5-17 mg/kg/min. for 10-15 minutes are necessary to cause moderate circulatory depression with tachycardia and lowered blood pressure. One unit of ACD blood would have to be infused every three to four minutes to a normal-sized patient to result in a lowering of blood pressure.[14]

Symptoms of paresthesias are observed more predominantly in smaller donors. Slow infusion of citrated blood adds to the general well-being and comfort of the donor. Increased amounts of citrate can be given to the donor unintentionally during excessive flushing of the extraction tubing in attempts at avoiding clotting at the venipuncture site.

Lymphocyte Depletion

Every intermittent-centrifugation plateletpheresis removes a substantial number of lymphocytes.[15] The donor's lymphocyte count is normal within a few hours to days following pheresis but the long-term safety of centrifugation pheresis still is unknown.[16,17] Some lymphocytes live

Table 3. — Citrate Concentrations in HES Citrate Solutions After Various Mixing Technics

Portion of Bottle	10 Minutes After 15 Seconds of Inversion	Time Following 30 Seconds of Forceful Agitation	
		5 min.	4 hours
Upper	0.34%	2.29%	2.0 %
Middle	2.60%	2.29%	2.29%
Lower	4.29%	2.29%	2.29%

Data from: Drescher, et al, Transfusion 18:89, 1978.

months and years, and so may become depleted by repeated pheresis since they are replaced more slowly. No side effects due to lymphocyte depletion have been recognized.

Clotting in the Extracorporeal Circuit

Sufficient anticoagulation for pheresis procedures should be prescribed in advance, and the ratio of anticoagulant to blood should be scrutinized during the procedure. Massive clotting has been observed in the bowl during intermittent-flow leukapheresis.[18] The mixture of citrate and HES can be incomplete for anticoagulation if not mixed vigorously for 30 seconds prior to the procedure. A simple inversion technic is not enough to provide an adequate homogeneous mixture. Inadequate mixing of citrate and HES may result in clotting after proceeding 45 to 60 minutes into the procedure (Table 3).

Hemolysis

Some red cells may be damaged during any mechanical manipulation of blood. This usually is negligible and not harmful to pheresis donors. However, the potential for hemolysis does exist wherever excessive flow restrictions may be found.

Lysis of donor red cells has been reported during intermittent-centrifugation pheresis using the Haemonetics Model 30.[19] For example, a twist or kink in the tubing leading from the bowl to the reinfusion bag can cause hemolysis (Fig 1). A visual check of the software during set-up

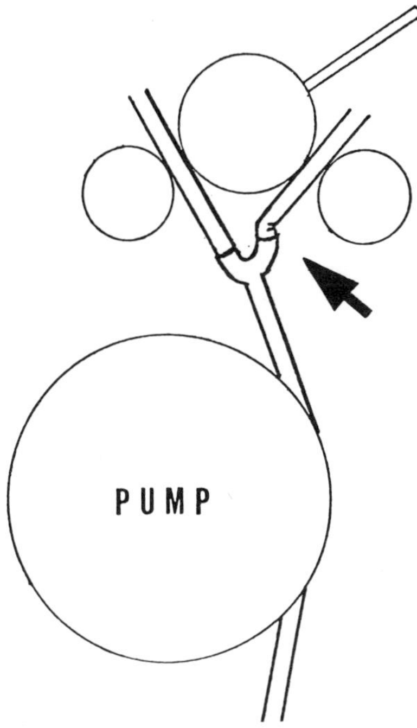

Fig 1. — Diagram of blood tube pathway of the Haemonetics Model 30 Blood Processor. The platelet-poor blood is pumped in an upward direction from the bowl to the reinfusion bag. The arrow designates the area where a twist or kink appeared, resulting in hemolysis.

and priming is essential. A slow bowl-emptying time may indicate obstruction. The presence of pink plasma in the bowl is a warning that lysis may have occurred. Once free hemoglobin is released into the circulation, it is observable as pink plasma in the following cycle. If this occurs these countermeasures are advised:

1. Discontinue blood withdrawal and infusion.
2. Keep a vein patent with isotonic saline.

3. Do not return any of the extracorporeal blood to the donor until the degree of hemolysis has been determined.
4. Alert the physician in charge.
5. Withdraw an anticoagulated sample from the donor and a clot sample from the reinfusion bag.
6. Centrifuge samples as an immediate visual confirmation of pink plasma. A comparator similar to that used in some frozen blood laboratories may provide an approximation of the amount of free hemoglobin present.
7. The donor should be encouraged to increase oral fluids and to report any subsequent dark brown, or black urine, abdominal or back pain, fever, chills, or any other unusual symptoms.
8. Urine samples from the donor should be collected at various intervals within the next 24 hours to document whether significant hemoglobinuria has developed.
9. Guidelines to indicate the degree of plasma hemoglobin that may be safely reinfused into the donor should be developed. Again, prevention and early recognition are the rule.

Air Embolism

Air embolism is the entry of air into the donor's circulation. Small amounts of air often enter the donor's venous system during any intravenous maneuver requiring manipulations and connections. Ordinarily, these are not harmful. There are no symptoms associated with small amounts of air in the circulation. Air can enter the donor venous circulation inadvertently during pheresis. Damage to the tubing may admit air and be pumped to the donor. Rapid infusion of blood by use of a blood pressure cuff around the Haemonetics Model-30 reinfusion bag is another potential source of air embolism and should be avoided. Death from air in the circulation may develop with as little as 5 ml/kg of body weight or 350 ml in a 70 kg individual.[20]

Large amounts of air may result in an "airlock" in the right ventricle, with air plugging the pulmonary vessels. Chest discomfort, difficult breathing, pallor, cyanosis, and hypotension may develop. A loud churning millwheel murmur may be heard with the stethoscope. The pain may be similar to other causes of chest pain such as angina, pneumothorax, dissecting aneurysm, pericarditis or esophagitis. However, the combination of the symptoms with obvious air in the tubing gives the immediate presumptive diagnosis. Countermeasures include:

1. Discontinue the infusion.
2. Maintain intravenous patency with isotonic saline.

3. Alert the pheresis physician.
4. Have the donor lie in a lateral position with left side down.
5. Apply nasal oxygen.
6. Monitor vitals.
7. Identify the site of air entry in the tubing.
8. Prevention is the rule. Pheresis personnel should observe every procedure continuously.

Abdominal Pain

Abdominal pain occurs rarely during filtration leukapheresis. However, this phenomenon seems to occur more frequently in female donors. Approximately 40 to 60 minutes into a pheresis procedure, the donor may complain of lower abdominal discomfort that has progressed from mild to severe cramping ("uterine-like" or "labor-like" pain) accompanied by the urge to defecate. The pain usually does not subside in less than 40 minutes after the procedure is discontinued, and may last for several hours. Countermeasures are:

1. Discontinue the procedure immediately.
2. Alert the physician.
3. Monitor vital signs.
4. A lateral position with knees bent may provide some symptomatic relief.

Of interest, Wiltbank, et al[21] reported that neither intravenous diazapam nor hydroxazine abolished the pain. Protamine afforded some relief in only three donors. Three donors subsequently donated by FL without incident.[21] Corticosteroid pretreatment appeared to have a protective effect.

Priapism

There have been two recently reported cases of priapism associated with FL. In both instances, the donor related that the problem occurred approximately 60 minutes following the start of FL. The cause is unknown. Both donors required surgical drainage.[22] In such cases the procedure should be terminated, the physician should be alerted, and a urological consultation should be obtained immediately.

Mechanical Difficulties

Mechanical difficulties occur on occasion and the pheresis staff should possess adequate knowledge of their equipment to be able to correct minor problems. Blown fuses, inadequate motor ventilation, and automatic clamp dysfunction are among some of the problems encountered.

Should a prolonged power failure occur, and emergency power is not available, the procedure must be terminated. Follow the manufacturer's instructions for the manual return of extracorporeal blood. For correctable instrument malfunctions and temporary power failures, remove the power plug and switch the instrument "off." Maintain an isotonic saline drip to prevent clotting until blood collection can be resumed.

In blood banking facilities it may be advantageous for staff to be familiar with the location of the house circuit-breaker box in case of circuit overload. This problem usually can be avoided by adequate preplanning in terms of the present and anticipated pieces of electrical equipment within the unit.

Hepatitis Risk to Donor and Staff

Blood spills are unavoidable in a pheresis unit and, therefore, they require attention to prevent possible hepatitis contamination of the staff and donors. Frequent hand-washing; the absence of eating, drinking, and smoking in work areas; and cleansing of machinery, table tops, and the donor couch immediately following blood spills, are recommended. A daily cleaning routine using 1:1 ratio of household bleach and water provides some measure of disinfection.

Postpheresis

Ordinarily, there are very few postpheresis problems. However, it is best to require the donor to remain at the blood center for an additional 20 to 90 minutes, depending upon the procedure. Before discharge, observe the venipuncture site to insure cessation of bleeding. If heparin is used without protamine, a pressure bandage should be applied and left in place for several hours. Ask the donor to restrict his/her physical activity for the remainder of the day.

Emergency Protocols

Written standard operating procedures explaining the management of reactions and emergencies are necessary. They should include emergency training, drills to be conducted regularly, and should state that CPR certification for all staff should be completed yearly. Serious consideration of appropriate medications and equipment for basic life support should be given. Phones should be labeled with emergency numbers. The possibility of an alarm system should be considered in order to obtain help, particularly if the pheresis unit is isolated. The management of severe reactions and emergencies, such as cardiac arrest, should be orderly and effective as a result of prior training and practice.

Records

Donor side effects, reactions and problems with the procedure should be adequately recorded on the procedure work record. In addition, all moderate and severe reactions should be reported in a separate "adverse reaction file." According to federal regulations adverse reactions reports regarding blood products arising as a result of blood collection must be maintained for five years.[23] Each incident should be well investigated and documented. A procedure for investigating adverse donor and recipient reactions must be part of the written standard operating procedures.[24] It is important to review adverse reactions regularly in order to better understand their nature and minimize risks to pheresis donors.

Summary

There are numerous side effects and adverse reactions that may accompany pheresis donations. However, they usually are mild and well tolerated by pheresis donors. In order to minimize the risks taken by the pheresis donor, the pheresis personnel must be thoroughly aware of them. In addition, excellent skills and constant alertness are needed for their prevention, early recognition, and management.

References

1. Engel GL: *Fainting.* Springfield, Charles C. Thomas, 1962, p 16.
2. Eastlund T, Kotwas A, Britten A: unpublished data.
3. Ebert RV, Stead Jr EA, Gibson JG: Response of Normal Subjects to Acute Blood Loss. *Arch Int Med* 68:578, 1941.
4. Caplan SN, Berkman EM: Protamine sulfate and fish allergy. *N Engl J Med* 295:172, 1976.
5. Mishler JM: Hydroxyethyl starch as an adjunct to leukocyte separation by centrifugal means: Review of safety and efficacy. *Transfusion* 15:449, 1975.
6. Thompson WL: Hydroxyethyl starch in blood substances and plasma expanders. Jamieson GA, Greenwalt TJ, Prog Clin Biolog Res vol 19 AR Liss Inc, 1978, pp 283-292.
7. Rock G, Wise P: Plasma expansion during granulocyte procurement: the accumulative effects of hydroxyethyl starch. *Blood* 52 suppl:203, 1978.
8. Ring J, Messmer K: Incidence and severity of anaphylactoid reactions to colloid volume substitutes. *Lancet* 1:466, 1977.

9. Schiffer, CA, Aisner J, Schmukler M, et al: The effect of hydroxyethyl starch on in vitro platelet and granulocyte function. *Transfusion* 15:449, 1975.

10. Mishler JM, Jones AW, Lowes B, et al: The utilization of a new strength citrate anticoagulant during centrifugal plateletpheresis. *Br J Haematol* 34:387, 1976.

11. Olson PR, Cox C, McCullough J: Laboratory and clinical effects of the infusion of ACD solution during plateletpheresis. *Vox Sang* 33:79, 1977.

12. Ladenson JH, Miller WV, Sherman LA: The relationship between physical symptoms, ECG, free calcium, and other blood chemistries in reinfusion with citrated blood. *Transfusion* 18:670, 1978.

13. Szymanski O: Ionized calcium during plateletpheresis. *Transfusion* 18:701, 1978.

14. Bunker JP, Bendixen HH, Murphy AJ: Hemodynamic effects of intravenously administered sodium citrate. *N Engl J Med* 266:372, 1962.

15. Segel GB, Lichtman MA, Gordon BR, et al: Plateletpheresis residues: a source of large quantities of human blood lymphocytes. *Transfusion* 16:495, 1976.

16. Lichtiger B, Trujillo JM: T and B lymphocytes in peripheral blood in normal donors after prolonged plateletpheresis. *Transfusion* 16:534, 1976, p 534.

17. Genco PV, Katz AJ: Redistribution of lymphocytes during discontinuous-flow plateletpheresis. *Blood* 52 (Suppl):298, 1978.

18. Drescher WP, Shih N, Hess K, et al: Massive extracorporeal blood clotting during discontinuous-flow leukapheresis. *Transfusion* 18:89, 1978.

19. Howard JE, Parkins HA: Lysis of donor RBC during plateletpheresis with a blood processor. *JAMA* 236:289-290, 1976.

20. Dexter L: *Pulmonary Embolism and Acute Cor Pulmonale in the Heart,* Nurst JW, Logue RB (eds). McGraw-Hill Co, 1970, p 1148.

21. Wiltbank TB, Nusbacher J, Higby DJ, et al: Abdominal pain in donors during filtration leukapheresis. *Transfusion* 17:159, 1977.

22. Dahlke MD, Shah SL, Sherwood WC, et al: priapism during filtration leukapheresis. *Transfusion,* 1978, in press.

23. Code of Federal Regulations 21, part 606.170, Food and Drug Administration, U.S. Department of Health, Education and Welfare, April, 1978.

24. Code of Federal Regulations 21, part 606.100 (b) (9), Food and Drug Administration, U.S. Department of Health, Education and Welfare, April, 1978.

Chapter 6

QUALITY ASSURANCE IN PHERESIS

Jeffrey McCullough, MD

Q UALITY CONTROL or quality assurance (QA), as it is often called, has been aggressively adopted by blood banks and transfusion services during the past several years. This was motivated partially by publication of the Food and Drug Administration (FDA) Good Manufacturing Practices for the collection, preparation, and transfusion of blood and components. QA is a difficult subject to discuss, even as applied to traditional aspects of blood collection and transfusion. Although it sometimes seems that blood banks are regulated and standardized beyond reasonable limits, there are many intentional vagaries in the QA required of blood banks. These vagaries are further clouded when one considers the many activities which could be considered part of quality assurance. There must be a knowledgeable staff who understand their duties and responsibilities and are kept abreast of changes in technics. Does this mean that hiring practices, preparation of procedure manuals, and staff continuing education are parts of QA? Many would answer, "Yes."

This discussion is included here because the issues become even more difficult when QA is applied to a relatively new technic like pheresis. Data defining the sources of variation or risks in pheresis are not as clear and available as some would like. Technics constantly change as efforts are made to obtain more cells in a shorter donation time. New instruments are developed. Finally, pheresis is different from ordinary blood donation in one important way; the blood bank is not only *removing* something, but *giving* foreign substances to the donors — saline and citrate solutions, drugs such as heparin, hydroxyethyl starch, dextran, steroids or protamine. Thus, pheresis involves all the risks of intravenous administration of drugs to normal individuals who go about their usual daily activities before and after the pheresis donation.

Considerations of QA in pheresis should include not only the composition of the final product and the usual attention to supplies, equipment, and records, but also attention to donor safety. QA procedures can be designed to monitor the *outcome* by testing the final product. In addition, it may be desirable to monitor the collection *process* to ensure a safe pheresis procedure. An analogy to production of ordinary components, such as platelet concentrate, can be made wherein the final product is monitored (pH, volume, platelet count), but the process also is monitored by testing centrifuge timers and speed. In pheresis it seems reasonable to monitor both the outcome (final product) and the process (pheresis procedure). However in QA, that which seems reasonable to one can seem unreasonable to another, so the approach described here is merely the author's personal opinion and should be taken in that light.

Personnel

Possibly the most important part of a high quality activity of any kind is good people. The hiring practices, job training and orientation, in-service education, performance evaluation, and general spirit and motivation are all important, but difficult to define. With a unique activity such as pheresis, selection and training of a good staff is an essential first step. A specific detailed training and orientation program should be available in each facility. If there is inadequate experience in the facility to provide training, personnel can be sent to established pheresis programs. A few days of training by a manufacturer's representative and/or attendance at a workshop is not sufficient, unless this can be supplemented by experienced pheresis personnel in the facility.

Records

As in other blood bank activities, maintenance of proper records is of utmost importance. The records should be legible and sufficiently comprehensive to allow reconstruction of the details of the pheresis procedure if necessary. The following pertinent data relating to each pheresis procedure should be recorded: the time the procedure was started and completed; blood-flow rates during the procedure; estimated total volume of blood processed; total volume retained (volume of product); volume of blood samples obtained; description and amount or dosage of all intravenous fluids and drugs administered to the donor before, during and after the procedure; lot numbers of all solutions; lot numbers of all plastic tubing sets; disposable bowls, or disposable blood separation chambers; and the unique donor identification number relating the pheresis procedure to the donor and the specific products obtained. If the collection facility uses more than one blood cell separator, each instrument should be assigned a code number and that number recorded to relate the particular procedure to a specific instrument. The identity of the individual carrying out the pheresis procedure should also be recorded along with an indication of whether an adverse reaction occurred during or after the procedure. Laboratory testing and processing of the product can be recorded on existing laboratory forms. If existing forms are not used, a new form should be developed so that all testing and handling of the unit is recorded in detail as for other blood products.

The Donor

Health History and Physical Examination

The donor's health affects the safety of the final product and the safety of the pheresis procedure itself. Thus, factors related to the donor are considered part of QA by some, but in this workshop they will be considered as part of donor selection and not discussed further here.

Laboratory testing of the donor (eg, CBC, platelet count, etc), although possibly more closely related to QA, also will be discussed as part of donor selection. Some laboratory and physical testing is necessary for donor selection, and accuracy of these tests should be monitored. Quality assurance procedures used in selection of whole blood donors, such as monitoring of hematocrit centrifuges, copper sulfate solutions, and sphygmomanometers should be carried out similarly for pheresis donors.

Labeling

Careful identification of the container and associated samples is the first step in accurate handling of the products. In this regard, pheresis products are not different from ordinary whole blood. Proper labels and a unique number should be applied to each container and associated tubes, preferably at the beginning of collection.

Venipuncture

A variety of needles and catheters is used for pheresis. Most experienced pheresis personnel have found some that seem to work better than others, although there is no universal agreement on ideal equipment. It seems advisable to maintain some record of the kind of needles or catheter used. This could be merely a general statement that all procedures done during a specified interval used certain needles.

Preparation of the venipuncture site usually is similar to the procedure used for collection of whole blood. Quality assurance of the solutions used and the adequacy of the skin preparation should be monitored, using procedures each blood bank has found suitable for whole blood collection. Recommendations for monitoring the venipuncture site include culturing the area with a moistened swab or touch plate,[1] or drawing blood into broth or ACD solution for culture.[2]

Volume Collected

As yet, there are no standards defining the volume of the final product or the maximum volume which can be removed from a donor during pheresis. During plasmapheresis, plasma removal is limited to 500 ml (600 ml if > 170 lbs.) during a 48-hour period, and 1000 ml (1200 ml if > 170 lbs.) per week. These might serve as guidelines, but need not necessarily be applied to cytapheresis, since the situation is different. The records should indicate the volume which has been retained from the donor.

Component Collection

It has been recommended that no more than 15% of the donor's estimated blood volume be extracorporeal at any time. This caveat is relevant only with the Haemonetics Model 30, but is disregarded frequently. With other instruments, the extracorporeal volume is stable and the volume of the final product is determined by the component collection rate.

Pheresis Procedure

There should be a written procedure describing the pheresis technic exactly, and good records should be kept indicating that the procedure was followed.

Pheresis Instruments

At present, there is no general policy from regulatory agencies or manufacturers regarding QA of pheresis instruments. At least five different instruments are available (Aminco Celltrifuge, Fenwal Leukapheresis Pump, Haemonetics Model 30, the original IBM Blood Cell Separator, and the IBM 2997 Blood Cell Separator). These instruments have different operating principles, and some have built-in monitors and alarms. It would seem prudent that a QA program be developed for each instrument that would periodically test: (1) any built-in monitors and alarms, and (2) parts of the instrument where malfunction could cause harm to the donor or product.

Single Donor Platelet Concentrates

Pheresis, today, is used to produce single donor platelets or granulocytes or a combination of both. Lymphocyte collection will not be considered here. At present, standards for pheresis products have not been established because: (1) there is continued modification of technics, (2) there is considerable variability from procedure to procedure, (3) different instruments may give different yields, and (4) the minimum clinically effective dose of granulocyte is not known. Since there are no AABB standards or FDA regulations defining a suitable pheresis platelet or granulocyte concentrate, each facility could set its own minimum and monitor the success in achieving this. Alternatively, the facility could set no minimum, but monitor performance and provide a description of that performance. I prefer the former.

Single Donor Platelet Concentrates

The Haemonetics Model 30 collects $2.8 - 5.5 \times 10^{11}$ platelets.[3-7] The number of platelets depends on the number of cycles of filling the bowl (Table 1), and the QA program should account for this. Our QA data indicate (for the small bowl) that almost 25% fewer platelets are collected when the Haemonetics is operated for six instead of eight cycles (Table 1). Some collections contain $<4.0 \times 10^{11}$ platelets. Since 75% of platelet concentrates prepared from ordinary units of whole blood

Table 1. — Quality Control Data for Platelet and Granulocyte Collection Using the Aminco Celltrifuge and the Haemonetics Model 30 (Small Bowl)

Instrument	No. Cycles	No. Tested	Platelets $\times 10^{11}$ Av	Range	No. Tested	Granulocytes $\times 10^{9}$ Av	Range
Celltrifuge	—	17	5.7	2.7 — 10.0	22	10.2	5.5 — 15.0
Haemonetics 30	8	37	6.6	4.0 — 10.0	11	9.6	3.7 — 22.1
	7	5	6.8	3.4 — 11.0	5	9.0	3.9 — 15.0
	6	4	5.1	3.7 — 7.7	23	6.9	3.1 — 12.1

should contain at least $.6 \times 10^{11}$ platelets, we felt that a plateletpheresis should be equivalent to at least a six-unit platelet concentrate. Thus, we selected 3.5×10^{11} platelets as a minimum to be contained in at least 75% of units tested. This has been achieved easily (Table 1).

The number of platelet concentrates which should be tested each month depends upon the number of procedures being done. In establishing a pheresis program, all plateletpheresis concentrates should be tested, to determine optimum technic and provide baseline data. Therefore, in a busy program, as few as 25% of units may be tested. If plateletpheresis is done infrequently, it is advisable to test all concentrates. If several instruments are used and staff members operate different instruments, the QA program should include all instruments so as to be representative of actual practice.

It is well known that platelet concentrates prepared from standard units of whole blood must maintain $pH > 6.0$ to remain effective after storage. It seems reasonable to apply this requirement to single-donor platelets. However, this may necessitate storage in a 2000 ml container to maintain pH, cell morphology, and recovery from osmotic stress.[8] Because of the variation in the number of platelets in different concentrates, the minimum volume necessary to maintain pH$>$6.0 is not known. It is difficult to measure pH since most concentrates will be transfused before the end of the storage period, and even if they are still available for testing at 24 or 48 hours, it is difficult to obtain samples without making the concentrates unusable. Since 3.5×10^{11} platelets is equivalent to approximately six random-donor units, a minimum volume of 300 ml may be necessary (6×50 ml).

Storage of Single Donor Platelet Concentrates

Despite widespread use of these platelet concentrates, there is not a single bit of direct information showing whether after storage they have normal intravascular survival or improve bleeding time. These platelets function normally immediately after collection.[9] Katz et al[8] found good maintenance of pH, morphology, and response to hypotonic stress after 24, and even 48, hours of storage. Anecdotal observations indicate that single-donor platelets stored up to 24 hours cause cessation of bleeding in thrombocytopenic patients. However, this is insufficient proof of efficacy to allow licensure of this product by FDA. It is presumed that temperature effects will be similar to random-donor platelet concentrate, and storage at room temperature will be preferable. Storage at room temperature of products collected in an "open" system with many connections may present a problem.

Presently, the FDA requires that red blood cells prepared in an open system be tested for sterility, but the American Association of Blood Banks does not. Sterility testing of pheresis products is difficult since most concentrates will be transfused and not available for testing after storage. The sterility of the system in use should be documented during its establishment; however, ongoing sterility testing does not seem practical, or may not be necessary. It is possible to flush the pheresis system with saline to obtain material for culture, if desired by the blood bank.

QA of Single-Donor Platelet Concentrates

The QA of the final product should involve a representative number, such as 25%, of all products. The platelet count and volume should be determined and the total number of platelets calculated (Table 2). At least 75% of the concentrates tested should contain a minimum of 3.5×10^{11} platelets and all concentrates should have a volume of at least 300 ml. These concentrates may be stored for up to 24 hours at room temperature, although data to support this are not available. At present, practical methods for determination of pH and sterility of stored units have not been developed, and may not be necessary.

Granulocyte Concentrates

Filtration leukapheresis (FL) produces more granulocytes than centrifuge leukapheresis (CL); however, it appears that a larger proportion of FL cells do not circulate following transfusion. FL granulocytes may easily be damaged during collection and may be affected by storage differently than are CL granulocytes. Thus, different requirements probably are necessary for QA of FL than CL. Because of this complexity, FL will not be considered further here.

Transfusion of as few as $.6 \times 10^{10}$ granulocytes has resulted in clinical benefit,[10] although 1.5×10^{10} has been recommended as the optimum dose.[11] When no steroids or HES are used, approximately $.5 \times 10^{10}$ granulocytes can be obtained with the Celltrifuge, and $.3 \times 10^{10}$ with the

---

Table 2. — Sample Calculation of Total Number of Platelets in Single-Donor Concentrate

---

Platelet count of concentrate $= 1,200,000/\mu 1$
Volume of concentrate $= 350$ ml
$1,200,000/\mu 1 = 1.2 \times 10^6/\mu 1$
$(1.2 \times 10^6/\mu 1) \times (350$ ml$) \times 1000$ ml$/\mu 1 = 4.2 \times 10^{11}$ total platelets

---

Haemonetics Model 30.[12] Use of either HES or steroids produces approximately 1×10^{10}; and use of both HES and steroids, produces upwards of 1.5×10^{10} granulocytes.[12] Transfusions containing less than 1×10^{10} granulocytes probably provide a barely adequate number of cells to be clinically effective in the adult.

There is a great deal of variability in the number of granulocytes obtained from different procedures and different donors. The sources of this variability are not well understood, but involve the donor granulocyte count and volume of blood processed through the pheresis instrument. Small veins, slow blood flow, and a low granulocyte count all contribute to poor granulocyte yields. Most published reports of leukapheresis include the mean or median number of granulocytes obtained, but not the range. Large samples of pheresis procedures may not include data on suboptimal or prematurely terminated procedures and the spectrum of results is not available in the literature. Thus, it is more difficult to establish minimum satisfactory granulocyte yields than platelet yields.

Transfusions containing less than 1×10^{10} granulocytes probably are

of only marginal clinical value in the adult. We would like to obtain this number of granulocytes in all concentrates, but have been unable to do so without using steroid treatment of the donors. Based upon our experience, we have arbitrarily chosen $.8 \times 10^{10}$ as the satisfactory granulocyte yield. The same approach as described earlier for platelets has been used, namely, that 75% of concentrates should contain the minimum number of granulocytes. This has been achieved with the Celltrifuge, but not with the Haemonetics Model 30, primarily because many donors are unable to tolerate eight cycles (Table 1). When only six cycles are done, the Haemonetics Model 30 does not provide a satisfactory product in our hands. Many published reports cite only optimum procedures and do not give an accurate picture of day-to-day reality. Steroid stimulation of donors prior to leukapheresis improves granulocyte yield and we have used a minimum of 1×10^{10} granulocytes as suitable for 75% of such collections.

Storage of Granulocyte Concentrate

The optimum storage conditions for granulocytes have not been defined. Granulocytes maintain the following in vitro functions nearly normal during the first 24 hours of storage, or even longer: bacterial and candida killing, phagocytosis, NBT reduction, oxygen consumption, and chemiluminescence.[13-15] Chemotactic response deteriorates earliest and to the greatest extent,[13-15] but can be better preserved by storage of granulocytes at room temperature instead of 4 C.[16] It may be important to maintain pH above 6.0 or 6.5[14,17] but since this is not yet established for granulocytes collected by CFCL or IFCL, it is not clear whether pH testing will be an important part of granulocyte concentrate QA. In one report, agitation during storage at room temperature was deleterious to chematatic response;[16] however the effects of agitation during storage cannot be considered settled. Unless there is comtamination with large numbers of organisms, the granulocytes should maintain sterility themselves. However, the necessity of routine sterility testing is not known. The effect of the type of plastic in the storage container, surface to volume ratio, cell concentrations, and many other variables, are not established. We prefer to transfuse granulocytes as soon as possible after collection, but allow storage of the concentrate for up to 24 hours at 20-24 C. However, at present, no studies of the in vivo effectiveness of stored granulocytes have been reported, so the clinical value of stored granulocytes to patients has not been established.

QA of Granulocyte Concentrates

QA of the final product should involve a representative number of all products, instruments, and staff. The granulocyte count and volume should be determined and the total number of granulocytes calculated. At least 75% of concentrates should contain $.8 \times 10^{10}$ granulocytes (1.0×10^{10} if steroids are used). The minimum volume has not been established. The hematocrit should be measured and the volume of red cells calculated. Concentrates may be stored at 4 C or room temperature for up to 24 hours, but should be transfused as soon as possible. It is not known whether routine pH and sterility testing is necessary.

Summary

QA of pheresis procedures and products is difficult and not well defined. The most important thing is that blood banks carrying out pheresis monitor their performance in an ongoing, organized way, so that changes in results or problems potentially dangerous to the donor or recipient will be identified.

References

1. *Technical Manual,* ed 7. Washington, DC, American Association of Blood Banks, 1977, p 288.
2. Myhre B: *Quality Control in Blood Banking.* New York, John Wiley & Sons, 1974, p 16.
3. Nusbacher J, Scher ML, MacPherson JL: Plateletpheresis using the Haemonetics Model 30 Cell Separator. *Vox Sang* 33:9, 1977.
4. Mishler JM, Janes AW, Lowes B, et al: The utilization of a new strength citrate anticoagulant during centrifugal plateletpheresis. I. Assessment of donor effects. *Br J Hematol* 34:387, 1976.
5. Katz AJ, Reiss FR, Houx JA: Redistribution of platelets during discontinuous flow platelet pheresis. *Vox Sang* 35:345, 1978.
6. Szymanski IO, Patti K, Kliman A: Efficacy of the Latham Blood Processor to perform platelet pheresis. *Transfusion* 13:405, 1978.
7. Tullis JL, Tinch RJ, Baudanza P, et al: Plateletpheresis in a disposable system. *Transfusion.* 11:368, 1971.
8. Katz A, Houx J, Ewald L: Storage of platelets prepared by discontinuous-flow centrifugation. *Transfusion* 18:220, 1978.
9. Slichter SJ: Efficacy of platelets collected by semi-continuous-flow centrifugation (Haemonetics Model 30). *Br J Hematol* 38:131, 1978.
10. Graw RG, Herzig G, Perry S, Henderson ES: Normal granulocyte transfusion therapy. *N Engl J Med* 287:367, 1972.
11. Higby DJ: Controlled prospective studies of granulocyte transfusion therapy. *Exp Hematol* 57:1977.
12. McCullough J: Leukapheresis and granulocyte transfusion, *CRC Crit Rev Clin Lab Sci Critical Reviews,* April, 1979, p 275.

13. McCullough J, Weiblen BJ: Relationship of granulocyte ATP to chemotatic response during storage. *Transfusion* (in press).
14. Steigbigel RT, Baum J, MacPherson JL, et al: Granulocyte bactericidal capacity and chemotaxis as affected by continuous-flow centrifuge and filtration leukapheresis, steroid administration, and storage. *Blood* 52:197, 1978.
15. Glasser L: Effect of storage on normal neutrophils collected by discontinuous-flow centrifugation leukapheresis. *Blood* 50:1145, 1977.
16. McCullough J, Weiblen BJ, Peterson PK, et al: Effects of temperature on granulocyte preservation. *Blood* 52:301, 1978.
17. McCullough J: Liquid preservation of granulocytes. *Transfusion,* in press.

Chapter 7

PRETRANSFUSION TESTING FOR PLATELET AND GRANULOCYTE THERAPY

Eugene M. Berkman, MD, and Jerome B. Orlin, MD

PHERESIS OF PLATELETS and granulocytes from normal donors has become relatively common in large regional blood programs and in many hospital-based blood banks. The pheresis procedures usually are accomplished using discontinuous[1] or continuous[2] centrifugation, and for granulocytes, only reversible nylon fiber adhesion.[3] These procedures are associated with increased donation time and loss of plasma and cellular elements in large numbers. The requirements for predonation testing of the donor and pretransfusion testing of the product differ from those applicable to red cell transfusion. Additionally, pretransfusion tests of serologic compatibility have not achieved the same level of sophistication for platelet and granulocyte transfusions as they have for red cell transfusion.

Donor Selection and Testing

General Considerations

The standards which apply to whole blood donation[4] should be followed when selecting pheresis donors. Under special circumstances, these requirements may be waived by a physician if the donated product is expected to be of particular value to the patient. Because aspirin and aspirin-containing medications may prolong the bleeding time significantly, donors who have ingested these medications prior to donation should not be heparinized unless their bleeding times are within normal limits.

Other pretransfusion tests applicable to whole blood should be carried out on platelet and granulocyte donors. Specifically, tests for hepatitis and unexpected antibodies should be completed prior to transfusion. Intravascular hemolysis due to passively transfused antibody[5] can be avoided if the principles that govern transfusion of plasma are applied to pheresis donors. Specific use of pheresis products with positive test results can be decided intelligently in each individual case, with appropriate balance of risks and benefits. Other tests on donors should follow guidelines for plasmapheresis[4] if donation is accomplished at frequent intervals over long periods of time. If donation frequency is similar to

89

that for whole blood, then tests to monitor plasma protein are not needed. More frequent donations, which may be associated with excessive plasma loss, require periodic serum protein determinations. An additional consequence of centrifugation cytopheresis procedures is the removal of cellular elements in large numbers, including lymphocytes[6] and stem cells.[7] The long-term effects of their removal are unknown and, although no known hazards have surfaced, guidelines are needed for limits on donation frequency.

Plateletpheresis: Selection of ABO- and Rh-Compatible Donors

The presence of A and B red cell antigens on platelets seems well established.[8,9] The results of in vivo studies investigating the effect of ABO compatibility on platelet recovery and survival have been conflicting. Studies have shown: (1) no direct effect of ABO incompatibility;[10] (2) decreased recovery but normal survival;[11] (3) an effect depending upon the degree of HLA compatibility[12] (ABO incompatibility effecting the 24-hour platelet increment of HLA selectively mismatched platelets, but not of HLA-compatible platelets); or (4) no effect on post-transfusion increments, regardless of the degree of HLA compatibility.[13] There are no data to suggest that ABO-incompatible platelet transfusions are clinically less effective than ABO-compatible platelets for treatment of the thrombocytopenic patient.

The transfusion of ABO-incompatible platelets, with the passive transfusion of anti-A and anti-B containing plasma, is a potential hazard. Severe intravascular hemolysis is a distinct possibility, although the magnitude of this problem in platelet transfusion therapy has not been evaluated completely. Several reports[14,15] indicate that hemolysis has occurred due to the passive transfusion of anti-A.

Table 1 is a summary of a retrospective analysis of our own experience during the past eight years. The total number of platelet units transfused is near 65,000 and respect of ABO compatibility was not part of the transfusion policy. A single case was reported to the blood bank because of clinical symptoms of severe rigor. The haptoglobin was low but within normal range, the plasma hemoglobin was just above normal limits. The urine hemosiderin was positive, but probably reflects mild asymptomatic intravascular hemolysis during the preceding weeks due to many units of ABO-incompatible platelet transfusions. All other cases were detected because the antiglobulin test became positive during subsequent pretransfusion testing for red cell transfusion. All cases involved anti-A reactions, two due to transfusion of A_1 cells into A_2 individuals. The antiglobulin test was positive with anti-IgG and, in some cases, anti-C3 antiserum.

This experience would indicate that clinical symptoms from transfusion of ABO-incompatible platelets are relatively unusual, but positive antiglobulin tests are more common. In fact, the incidence may be even greater than indicated by these cases, since no attempt was made to ascertain the actual incidence. No one has documented a consistent effect of passively-transfused anti-A on red cell survival or increased transfusion requirements in these patients, but this may exist. ABO compatibility is desirable to avoid the complications of passively-transfused antibody, and would be considered ideal. Logistics of platelet support generally preclude this ideal. Clinical data indicate that serious complications are

Table 1. — Positive Antiglobulin Tests In Patients Who Receive ABO-Incompatible Platelet Transfusions

Diagnosis	Age/Sex	ABO Type	Heat Eluate	Antiglobulin Test	
				Anti-IgG	Anti-C3
ALL	3/M	A_1	Anti A_1	+	+
ALL	5/F	A_2B	Anti A_1*	+	+
AML	15/F	A_2	Anti A_1*	+	'
AML	17/M	A_1	Anti A_1	+	'
Hemorrhage	42/F	A_1	Anti A_1	+	+
AML	57/M	A_1	Anti A_1	+	'
CAD	46/M	A_1	Anti A_1	+	+
CML	64/M**	A_1	Anti A_1	+	+
MM	73/F	A_1	Anti A_1	+	'
AML	74/M	A_1B	Anti A_1	+	'

* Transfused with A_1 cells (2 units)
** Symptomatic (Severe Rigors) (Haptoglobin 75mg%)
(Plasma Hgb 5.6mg%) (Urine Hemosiderin +)

rare, and ABO-incompatible transfusions should not be withheld. If a positive antiglobulin test develops in the recipient, continued platelet support probably should be ABO-compatible, and, in some instances, the transfusion of washed group O cells may be indicated.

Rh antigens are not present on platelets,[16] but red blood cell contamination of platelet concentrates requires consideration of donor-recipient Rh type if Rh immunization is to be avoided. In one report,[17] immunosuppressed patients were shown to have a lower incidence of Rh immunization than normal, but the role of ABO incompatibility on Rh sensitization is difficult to evaluate in this study. Rh immune globulin could be administered to prevent sensitization if Rh-positive concentrates were transfused to an Rh-negative recipient in an emergency situation. The presence of Rh antibody does not preclude renal transplantation[18] or bone marrow transplantation.[19] Consideration of Rh type is important only for the consequences of immunization, since recovery and survival of transfused platelets is not effected by Rh incompatibility.[10,20]

Leukapheresis: Selection of ABO- and Rh-Compatible Donors

In selecting granulocyte donors, ABO and Rh must also be considered. The usual methods of granulocyte procurement result in erythrocyte contamination and most published studies have used ABO-compatible donors routinely to avoid transfusion of ABO-incompatible red cells.[21-29] In some centers where HLA identity is considered important, ABO lines are commonly ignored and the risk accepted (Hester, JP: Workshop Am Soc Clin Histocompat Testing. San Diego, Calif., May, 1979). Although no difference in posttransfusion granulocyte increments has been reported between ABO-compatible and ABO-incompatible granulocyte transfusions,[30] one hour posttransfusion increments have been shown to be significantly lower in HLA-matched, ABO-mismatched granulocyte transfusions, than in HLA- and ABO-matched transfusions.[31] Whether this reflects the presence of ABO antigens on leukocytes is not known, and controversy over their presence on granulocytes exists.[32,33] The clinical effectiveness of ABO-matched versus ABO-mismatched granulocytes remains undetermined. Transfusion of ABO-incompatible plasma has been discussed. Current methods of granulocyte collection mandate ABO compatibility, unless exceptions are justified for specific reasons. Rh antigens are not present on granulocytes,[33,34] and transfusion considerations regarding Rh immunization depends upon red blood cell contamination and the risks of sensitization.

Recipient Selection and Testing

General Considerations

Technologic developments have made platelet and granulocyte transfusion therapy a reality and there is increasing utilization of these components. Questions regarding the detection and identification of antigen-antibody systems have arisen. Efforts to develop compatibility tests which will avoid the occasional serious transfusion reactions seen, and also predict the ability of transfused components to survive and function normally, have met with limited success. First, no single, simple test has been shown capable of detecting all antibody-containing serums. Second, in vitro serologic tests are not available which will predict, with a high degree of accuracy, the survival of transfused components. Patients with severe thrombocytopenia, with or without hemorrhage; patients with quantitative platelet defects and bleeding; and patients with severe neutropenia and infection are the usual recipients of platelet and granulocyte transfusions. Red cell compatibility testing is not required for platelet transfusions, since platelet concentrates generally contain very small numbers of contaminating red cells. Granulocyte concentrates, however, do contain significant numbers of red blood cells and, in general, should be serologically-compatible. The problems of ABO incompatibility have been discussed above.

Occasionally, red cell antibody may be present in the recipient and compatible donors are difficult to find. In these instances, the decision to transfuse incompatible red cells must be made by a physician after consideration of the expected risks and benefits. We have transfused Rh1(D)-incompatible and P1-incompatible granulocyte concentrates without clinical signs or symptoms. The importance of red cell antigens present on platelets and granulocytes, and their corresponding antibodies present in recipients, is unknown.

Platelet Compatibility Tests

Current technics to detect antiplatelet antibody-containing serums include both serologic and metabolic methods. The serologic tests include antiglobulin consumption,[35] complement fixation,[36,37] thromboagglutination,[38] lymphocytotoxicity, immunofluorescence, and an ^{125}I anti-immunoglobulin test. Methods which depend upon changes in metabolic function of platelets in the presence of antibody include serotonin-release assays, measurements of Platelet Factor 3 activity and platelet aggregation. Only the basic principles of tests used by investigators to perform compatibility tests for platelet transfusion are outlined:

Lymphocyte Cytotoxicity Test (LCT): In this test,[39] panel lymphocytes are prepared from whole blood by defibrination with glass beads, and then separation on a ficoll hypaque gradient. Following aspiration and centrifugation of the lymphocyte layer, contaminating red cells usually are removed by lysis with ammonium chloride. The lymphocytes are suspended in media and the concentration is adjusted to 2 to $2.5 \times 10^3/\mu\mathrm{l}$. Cells can be used directly, frozen in vials,[40] or frozen under oil in typing trays.[41] Dimethylsulfoxide (DMSO) is used as a cryoprotective agent. For the detection of lymphocytotoxic antibody, test serum is added to the fresh or thawed lymphocytes and incubated at room temperature for 30 minutes. Rabbit complement is then added and the mixture incubated for 60 minutes at room temperature. Excess complement is removed and

0.4% trypan blue is added. After 10 minutes incubation at room temperature, trypan blue is removed by flipping and the cells are resuspended in barbitol buffer. The wells are read with an inverted microscope. In the presence of lymphocytotoxic antibody, appropriate panel cells are unable to exclude trypan blue. Eosin dye can be used also.

Immunofluorescence: Immunofluorescent tests for the detection of antibody have been described recently. In one method,[42] a platelet suspension is prepared from whole blood collected in EDTA. The platelets are washed and then incubated at room temperature with a 1% paraformaldehyde solution (PFA) to prevent the nonspecific uptake of protein. The PFA-fixed platelets are incubated with test serums at 37 C for 30 minutes, washed, and then incubated with fluorescein isothiocynate-labeled antiglobulin serum (FITC-labeled IgG serum). The platelet suspension is then examined with a fluorescent microscope. For detection of complement on the cell surface, the washed platelets are treated similarly, but incubated with FITC-labeled anti-C3. The sensitivity, specificity, and reproducibility of the tests compare favorably with other methods and have the advantage of detecting either immunoglobulin or complement at the cell surface. An immunofluorescence test which does not require platelet fixation with PFA has been published, also.[43]

Platelet Serotonin Release: This test is reported to be capable of detecting autoimmune, isoimmune, or drug-induced antibodies.[44,45] Platelets are labeled with ^{14}C serotonin, and washed, resuspended, and added to test plasma. The mixture is incubated at 37 C for 45 minutes, centrifuged, and the radioactivity in an aliquot of the supernate is measured in a scintillation counter. Because labeled platelets, even in the presence of normal serum, will release serotonin in a time-dependent fashion, the reaction times are critical and a series of normal controls are required. Both complement-fixing and noncomplement-fixing antibodies are detected.

Platelet Factor 3 Activity: The test[46,47] depends upon the principle that Platelet Factor 3 activity measurably increases with platelet injury. In one method[46] platelet-rich plasma is incubated with heat-inactivated test serum at 37 C for 60 minutes. The mixture is stirred frequently, and an aliquot is withdrawn at 15-minute intervals. A Stypven time is performed on the aliquot, and platelet factor 3 activity is measured as a decrease in the Stypven time from normal controls. The test is considered positive if the test serums shorten the Stypven time by 10 seconds compared to normal controls. The test has been shown to be positive in cases of quinidine-induced thrombocytopenia, but is negative in autoimmune thrombocytopenia. Platelet Factor 3 activity may also be increased by nonimmunological mechanisms of platelet injury.

Platelet Aggregometry: In this test,[48] platelet-rich plasma is prepared from citrated or heparinized whole blood, and test serum is inactivated by heating at 56 C for 30 minutes (to remove traces of thrombin). The platelet rich-plasma is stirred, and changes in optical density are recorded as test serum is added. The presence of isoantibodies is detected by a marked decrease in optical density of the mixture. The reaction time, the interval from the addition of serum to a decrease of 0.1 optical density units, may be used to quantitate changes in antibody titer, or to compare potency between different serums. The test appears to have a sensitivity comparable to complement fixation. While isoimmune and drug-induced antibodies are detected, autoimmune antibodies are not.

^{125}I Anti-Immunoglobulin Test: An ^{125}I anti-immunoglobulin test has been developed.[49] In this test, human IgG is coupled to CNBr-activated Sepharose 4B and used to immunoabsorb anti-IgG from commercially available reagents. The anti-IgG is eluted with HC1 glycin buffer, concentrated, and labeled with ^{125}I. A platelet suspension is incubated with heat-inactivated test serum for 30 minutes at 37 C and then washed. The platelets are then incubated with ^{125}I anti-IgG for 20 minutes at room temperature. After washing, the radioactivity of the platelet pellet is determined and expressed as a percent of total radioactivity. The test does not depend upon the viability of test platelets, nor on the complement-fixation properties of antibody.

The Role of HLA and Platelet-Specific Antigens

Initial reports described the good results obtained from the transfusion of platelets from HLA-compatible siblings to patients with aplastic anemia who had become refractory to random-donor platelets.[50] In subsequent studies, this observation was extended to the transfusion of platelets from unrelated HLA-compatible donors.[51,52] The observation was made that the presence of selected donor antigens not present in the recipients may not have an adverse effect on the platelet response. This was confirmed in transfusion between an HLA-A12-positive donor and an HLA-A12-negative recipient.[53]

Because of the magnitude of establishing an adequate HLA donor bank, many other clinical studies have been performed with a goal of assessing the minimum degree of HLA compatibility required to achieve satisfactory results.[13,52,54,55] It has been reported that specific antigens known to be crossreactive may be selectively mismatched without adverse effect,[56,57] and it has been estimated that the use of selected mismatches could allow for a 20% decrease in the size of a histocompatible platelet-transfusion donor pool. In contrast, the transfusion of platelets from an

HLA-A2-positive donor to a patient with anti-HLA-A2 may lead to rapid in vivo platelet destruction.[58] Since HLA-A2 is one of the most immunogenic of the HLA antigens,[59] approximately one third of multi-transfused, HLA-A2-negative patients will develop cytotoxic antibody.[60]

While there has been success in the management of selected cases with the use of HLA-compatible platelets, it has become apparent that not all HLA-compatible platelet transfusions achieve the degree of success expected. Disappointing results are seen in at least 20%-40% of platelet transfusions completely matched for the HLA-A and HLA-B locci.[61,62] There are data that there may be, in fact, little or no correlation between HLA compatibility and a successful transfusion.[63] The possible role of the C locus in this regard has been investigated, but compatibility in this system does not appear to influence survival,[61] and the existence of other relevant platelet antigen systems is presumed.

Of the known platelet-associated antigens,[65] $P1^{A1}$ appears to be the only one thus far identified which has been implicated in clinical immune disease. Anti-$P1^{A1}$ has been shown to be responsible for some cases of neonatal thrombocytopenia, as well as some cases of posttransfusion purpura. The antibody involved in these cases, however, is serologically different from other isoimmune anti-$P1^{A1}$ antibodies in that it is not complement-fixing, but is demonstrated by "blocking" tests of complement fixation.[66] Transfusion of serum containing complement fixing, anti-$P1^{A1}$ to $P1^{A1}$-positive patient will result in prolonged thrombocytopenia.[67] Reports of problems in platelet transfusion therapy due to anti-$P1^{A1}$ could not be found.

Refractoriness and Compatibility Testing

Refractoriness to platelet transfusions usually has been defined as the lack of an adequate rise in platelet count. Appropriate treatment of the refractory patient has been problematic, and most centers empirically have chosen one of the methods outlined above to select "compatible" platelet donors. Only recently have studies attempted to critically evaluate and compare these tests from the standpoint of their adequacy to predict response to platelet therapy. These clinical studies* have focused on the lymphocytotoxicity test, Platelet Factor 3 assay, serotonin release assay, platelet aggregometry, and the platelet fluorescence test. Data are contradictory. The accuracy of the lymphocytotoxicity assay to predict the results of transfusion has been shown in one series to be as high as 70%.[69] It also has been shown to be useful in predicting com-

---

*12, 13, 43, 54, 56, 61, 63, 64, 68.

patibility in selectively-HLA-mismatched recipient pairs, even though it was not helpful in predicting compatibility in fully HLA-matched transfusions.[55] In contrast, others have found a 70% incidence of false-positives and 40% incidence of false-negative tests.[70] These investigators could find no correlation between a positive lymphocytotoxicity test and an incompatible transfusion, regardless of the extent of HLA compatibility.

In another study, applying the results of a platelet fluorescence test to HLA-matched, lymphocytotoxic-test-negative, donor-recipient pairs did reduce the number of unsuccessful transfusions to 7%, and these "false-negative" fluorescence tests occurred only in two and three antigen mismatches.[43] The antibody specificity that accounts for the "true positive" test in this system is not known and further investigation is required to explain and confirm these results. As with lymphocytotoxicity, the data regarding the effectiveness of assays of Platelet Factor 3 release, platelet serotonin release, and aggregometry to predict response to platelet transfusion are contradictory.[71] Table 2 contains a summary of compatibility test results.

Regardless of the type of compatibility test under investigation, results have been evaluated on the basis of either posttransfusion platelet increments, platelet survival, or both. While this is convenient, it may be that these parameters are sufficient, but not necessary for the definition of a clinically effective platelet transfusion.[72] There is good evidence that in the untransfused patient, the incidence of hemorrhage increases with the degree of thrombocytopenia.[73] It also has been shown, however, that patients transfused prophylactically have a lower incidence of hemorrhage than untransfused patients, even if there is not a statistically significant difference between the platelet counts of the two groups.[74] It would appear from these studies that platelet count increments may not be the best way to evaluate the success of prophylactic platelet transfusion, and that many patients (perhaps the vast majority) may be treated successfully with random-donor or single-donor platelets,[75] even though posttransfusion increases in platelet counts are not evident.

Granulocyte Compatibility Tests

Granulocyte antigen systems and antibody interactions have been defined only recently. The serologically defined granulocyte antigens include granulocyte specific antigens, antigens shared with other leukocytes (ie, HLA antigens) and antigens shared with red blood cells. No single test method appears adequate to detect all cases of granulocyte antigen-antibody interactions. Methods published to date include agglutination, dye exclusion, and indirect immunofluorescence, as well as methods which measure either the neutrophil opsonizing effect of antibody-containing serum or its effects on neutrophil metabolic functions. A complement-fixation method[76] and an antibody-dependent, lymphocyte-mediated granulocyte cytotoxicity test[77] have also been described. They have not been used for clinical compatibility testing and will not be described further.

Microgranulocyte Cytotoxicity: The principle of this test[78] is similar to the previously described lymphocytotoxicity test. A granulocyte suspension is obtained by dextran sedimentation of heparinized blood followed by separation over ficoll hypaque. Following centrifugation and aspiration of the supernant containing platelets and lymphocytes, contaminating red cells are removed as described above. Because viable granulocytes adherent to the walls of the typing trays appear as dead cells, granulocyte

Table 2. — Platelet Compatibility Tests, Predictive Value and False Negative Results

Test	Predictive Value (%)	False Negatives (%)
a) LCT	30–70	23–30
b) Fluorescence	93	10
c) Serotonin release	47–88	60
d) Factor 3 activity	46	76
e) Aggregometry	59–90	12–83
f) ^{125}I anti-immunoglobulin	no data	no data

adherence must be inhibited. This can be accomplished by incubation at 37 C for 30 minutes with 0.1% iodoacetomide.

A modification of this technic has used cytochalasin B solubolized in DMSO (5μg/ml).[79] The iodoacetomide or cytochalasin-B-treated granulocytes are then incubated with the test serum at room temperature for 30 minutes in microtitre trays. Rabbit complement which has been absorbed with human red cells at 4 C for one hour to remove heterologous granulocyte cytotoxins, is added and the system is incubated for 60 minutes. Excess complement is removed. Trypan blue (0.4%) is added and incubated for 10 minutes. Following removal of excess trypan blue, the cells are resuspended in barbitol buffer and read with an inverted microscope. The percent of cytolysis is assessed with eosin or trypan blue exclusion. Another modification of this system has included the use of a discontinuous double-density ficoll hypaque gradient for granulocyte separation.[80] A two-stage microcytotoxicity test has been described also.[81] In this method, serum and cells are incubated for 30 minutes at 4 C in the presence of absorbed rabbit complement. Following the addition of complement, the suspension is incubated at 22 C for 3 hours. Cytotoxicity is determined by the degree of eosin dye exclusion.

Indirect Immunofluorescence: In this test,[82] coating of neutrophils by antineutrophil antibody is detected by the use of fluorescein-labeled anti-human Ig serum. Granulocytes are prepared from EDTA-treated whole blood by dextran sedimentation, followed by separation on a ficoll hypaque gradient. Nonspecific uptake of the fluorescein isothiocynate-labeled antihuman immunoglobulin serum (FITC-labeled Ig serum) is prevented by prefixing granulocytes with 1% paraformaldehyde at room temperature for five minutes. The cells are washed, incubated with an equal amount of test serum for 30 minutes at 37 C, and then washed again. The cells are then incubated with FITC-labeled rabbit antihuman Ig serum for 30 minutes at room temperature. The cells are washed and examined with a fluorescence microscope. The observed fluorescence is a measure of antibody activity in the serum.

Leukoagglutination: A variety of methods[83] for the detection of leuko-agglutinating activity in serum have been published. All depend upon the presence of EDTA as a chelating agent, although the mechanism of this dependence is not known. Because of problems with reproducibility, and the quantity of reagents required with macroagglutination technics, microagglutination technics have been developed.[84,85] In one method,[84] a buffy coat (granulocytes and mononuclear cells) is prepared from whole blood by defibrination with glass beads and centrifugation. Contaminating red cells are agglutinated with anti-H lectin or anti-A,B antibody. Following centrifugation, to remove the red cell aggregates, and several washing procedures, the leukocytes are resuspended in 10% EDTA and granulo-cyte donor serum. Microliter quantities of cells and test serum are incubated in microtiter trays at 37 C and examined for agglutination with an inverted phase microscope after 5 or 18 hours.

A capillary agglutination technic has been developed[86] which may be more sensitive than microagglutination. In this test, the presence of appropriate antileukocyte antibody in test serum prevents the dissociation of sensitized granulocytes. This is measured as the length of cell "stream" formation when the cell pellet dissociates by gravity in capillary tubes at a 45° angle. This method may detect both granulocyte-specific and HLA antibodies.

Neutrophil Opsonization: In this method,[87] the presence of antineutro-phil antibodies in serum is measured by the ability of the test serum to promote neutrophil ingestion by alveolar macrophages and the simul-taneous conversion of nitroblue tetrazolium to formazan. Neutrophils are obtained by density gradient centrifugation and rabbit macrophages are obtained by tracheal lavage from rabbits treated with complete Freund's adjuvant. Neutrophils are sensitized with heat inactivated test serum for 30 minutes at 25 C and then incubated with the macrophage suspension and nitroblue tetrazolium. After incubation at 37 C the reaction is stopped with 1mM N-ethylmaleimide. After centrifugation, the cells are extracted with dioxane and the quantity of nitroblue tetrazolium reduced to nitroblue tetrazolium formazan is measured spectrophotometrically.

Inhibition of Phagocytosis-Associated Hexose Monophosphate Shunt Activity: In this technic,[88] donor granulocytes are incubated at 37 C for 30 minutes with frozen test serum and fresh donor serum. The suspension is then incubated for an additional 60 minutes with a solution containing glucose-1-^{14}C and polystrene latex particles. The amount of $^{14}CO_2$ produced is measured by absorption onto KOH-soaked filters and counted in a liquid scintillation counter. The counts from a control serum are compared with the test serum and antibody activity is measured as a decrease in $^{14}CO_2$ production.

Role of Compatibility Testing, HLA, and Granulocyte-Specific Antigens

All of these methods are capable of identifying certain antibody-containing serums. Their specificities and sensitivities vary greatly, however, and studies comparing one method with all others are lacking. While it appears that indirect immunofluorescence may be more sensitive than granulocytotoxicity or leukoagglutination, the usefulness of this test, or indeed of any other of these tests, for compatibility testing prior to transfusion has not been demonstrated. Although clinical studies reported thus far have used a variety of "compatibility" tests, data supporting the role of any of these as routine pretransfusion tests are controversial.

Granulocyte-specific antigens, designated NA1, NA2, NB1, NC1, and ND have been described, and antibodies to these antigens have developed from neonatal sensitization, platelet transfusion, and granulocyte transfusions.[83] It is certain that these antibodies, as well as antibodies to other as yet uncharacterized antigens, are causative in some febrile transfusion reactions.

The extent to which an incompatibility in these systems, as indicated by the presence in the recipient of leukoagglutinating or granulocytotoxic antibodies directed toward donor granulocytes, causes adverse clinical effects, is controversial. Early studies[89,90] using granulocytes from donors with chronic myelogenous leukemia showed that posttransfusion increments and the percentage of posttransfusion-recovered granulocytes were markedly decreased in patients with alloantibodies directed against donor granulocytes, as compared to recipients without alloantibodies. Antibodies were detected as leukoagglutinins, although most serums also contained lymphocytotoxic antibodies. Furthermore, these investigators found a significantly higher incidence of transfusion reactions in alloimmunized recipients and presented data to suggest that in vitro phagocytosis and bacterial killing was also impaired by antibody-containing serum.

In animal studies,[91] one-hour posttransfusion increments and chemotaxis were decreased when granulocytes were transfused to granulocytopenic, alloimmunized dogs, compared to unimmunized animals. In this study, lymphocytotoxic antibody was present, as well as granulocytotoxic and leukoagglutinating antibody. In contrast, the results of 187 granulocyte transfusions in 19 patients demonstrated no correlation between the presence of alloantibodies (leukoagglutinating, granulocytotoxic, or lymphocytotoxic) and either granulocyte recovery or transfusion reactions.[92]

Even less is known regarding the nature of HLA-associated granulocyte antigens. Based upon absorption experiments, it seems certain that these antigens are present on granulocytes. Their representation on the membrane, however, does not appear sufficient to support a complement-dependent, granulocytotoxicity assay.[33] The clinical importance of HLA compatibility for granulocyte transfusion is unknown. Attempts to correlate HLA compatibility with posttransfusion granulocyte increments, transfusion reactions, and patient survival have been made in only a limited number of studies. A correlation between HLA compatibility and posttransfusion increments or survival has been reported,[31,93,94] but this finding has not been confirmed.[23,25]

Other clinical studies have reported the effectiveness of granulocyte transfusion therapy without presenting data regarding alloimmunization of recipients.[21,22,24,30] Donors usually were ABO-compatible, but were otherwise chosen at random, and no effort was made to use family members or HLA-compatible sibs. The results obtained in these studies are generally the same as in those studies utilizing a variety of pretransfusion tests and suggest that such testing, with current technics, does not improve results. The use of these tests as predictors of alloimmunization is further complicated by the presence of non-HLA lymphocytotoxic antibodies[95] and both warm and cold reactive granulocytotoxic antibodies[96,97] in patients with a variety of diseases.

There is no agreement upon the ability of the lymphocytotoxicity, leukoagglutination, or granulocytotoxicity crossmatch to predict transfusion reactions. These reactions commonly include fever, chills, mild dyspnea and agitation.[98] Less commonly, severe dyspnea, hypotension and the development of pulmonary infiltrates occur.[99] Although it has been suggested that these reactions may result from the presence of leukocyte alloantibodies,[27,93] there are data to the contrary. A recent report[92] found antileukocyte antibodies in 52% of granulocyte transfusion recipients, but no statistically significant relationship between the presence of antibody and neutrophil recovery or the incidence of transfusion reaction. Furthermore, serious reactions have occurred after transfusion of HLA-identical leukocytes to "compatible" recipients.[98]

Conclusion

The value of pretransfusion compatibility testing prior to platelet therapy, given current technics, is still open to question. For those patients receiving cytotoxic chemotherapy in whom thrombocytopenia is predictable and of limited duration, the transfusion of previously frozen autologous platelets offers a way to circumvent alloimmunization and the need for subsequent compatibility testing.[100] For other alloimmunized patients, available data suggest that many may respond clinically to random donor platelets despite lack of platelet increments. For those patients who do not respond clinically to random donor units, further response may be achieved by transfusion of HLA-matched single donor platelets or occasionally, even non-HLA-matched platelets.

Recommendations regarding a pretransfusion granulocyte compatibility test cannot be made. Further investigations are needed before compatibility testing will be able to improve the safety and efficacy of granulocyte transfusions.

Acknowledgement

This work was supported by National Institutes of Health Grant No. RO1 AM21027-01.

References

1. Tullis JL, Tinch RJ, Baudanza P, et al: Plateletpheresis in a disposable system. *Transfusion* 11:368-377, 1971.
2. Freireich EJ, Judson G, Levin RH: Separation and collection of leukocytes. *Cancer Res* 25:1516-1520, 1965.
3. Djerassi I, Kim JS, Mitrakul C: Filtration leukopheresis for separation and concentration of transfusable amounts of normal human granulocytes. *J Med (Basel)* 1:358-364, 1970.
4. *Standards for Blood Banks and Transfusion Services,* ed 9. Washington, DC, American Association of Blood Banks, 1978.
5. Morse EE: Interdonor incompatibility as a cause of reaction during granulocyte transfusion. *Vox Sang* 35:215-218, 1978.

6. Segel GB, Lichtman MA, Gordon BR, et al: Plateletpheresis Residues: A source of large quantities of human blood lymphocytes. *Transfusion* 16:455-459, 1976.

7. Weiner RS, Richman CM, Yankee RA: Semicontinuous flow centrifugation for the pheresis of immunocompetent cells and stem cells. *Blood* 49:391-397, 1977.

8. Dausset J, Malinvand G: Normal and pathological platelet agglutinins investigated by means of the shaking method. *Vox Sang* 4:204-213, 1954.

9. Coombs RRA, Bedford D: The A and B antigens on human platelets demonstrated by means of mixed erythrocyte-platelet agglutination. *Vox Sang* 5:111-115, 1955.

10. Shulman NR: Immunological considerations attending platelet transfusion. *Transfusion* 6:39-49, 1966.

11. Aster RH: Effect of anticoagulant and ABO incompatibility on recovery of transfused human platelets. *Blood* 26:732-743, 1965.

12. Duquesnoy RJ, Hackbarth S, Tomasulo PA, et al: Role of ABO compatibility and lymphocytotoxicity crossmatching in platelet transfusion therapy of alloimmunized thrombocytopenic patients, abstracted. *Transfusion* 18:639, 1978.

13. Tosato G, Appelbaum FR, Deisseroth AB: HLA-matched platelet transfusion therapy of severe aplastic anemia. *Blood* 52:846-854, 1978.

14. Zoes C, Dube VE, Miller HJ, et al: Anti-A_1 in the plasma of platelet concentrates causing a hemolytic reaction. *Transfusion* 17:29-32, 1977.

15. Lundberg WB, McGinniss MH: Hemolytic transfusion reaction due to anti-A_1. *Transfusion* 15:1-9, 1975.

16. Gurevitch J, Nelken D: Studies on platelet antigens III. Rh-Hr antigens in platelets. *Vox Sang* 5:82-93, 1957.

17. Goldfinger D, McGinniss MH: Rh-incompatible platelet transfusion risks and consequences of sensitizing immunosuppressed patients. *N Engl J Med* 284:942-944, 1971.

18. Hamburger J, Crosnier J, Dormont J, et al (eds): *Renal Transplantation, Theory and Practice*. Baltimore, Williams and Wilkins Co, 1972, p 47.

19. Berkman EM, Caplan SN: Engraftment of Rh-positive marrow in a recipient with Rh antibody. *Transplant Proc* 9:215-218, 1977.

20. Pfisterer H, Thierfelder S, Kottusch H, et al: Untersuchung menschlicker thrombocyten auf Rhesus-antigene durch abbaustudien in vivo nach ^{51}Cr-markierung. *Klin Wochenschr* 45:519-522, 1967.

21. Berkman EM, Eisenstaedt RS, Caplan, SN: Supportive granulocyte transfusions in the infected severely neutropenic patient. *Transfusion* 18:693-700, 1978.

22. Hershko C, Naparstek E, Eldor A, et al: Granulocyte transfusion therapy: a clinical trial in patients with acute leukemia and sepsis. *Vox Sang* 34:129-135, 1978.

23. Higby DJ, Yates JW, Henderson ES, et al: Filtration leukapheresis for granulocyte transfusion therapy. *N Engl J Med* 292:761-766, 1975.

24. Alavi JB, Root RK, Djerassi I, et al: A randomized clinical trial of granulocyte transfusions for infection in acute leukemia. *N Engl J Med* 296:706-711, 1977.

25. Herzig RH, Herzig GP, Graw RG, et al: Successful granulocyte transfusion therapy for gram-negative septicemia. *N Engl J Med* 296:701-705, 1977.

26. Boggs DR: Transfusion of neutrophils as prevention or treatment of infection in patients with neutropenia. *N Engl J Med* 290:1055-1062, 1974.

27. Goldman JM: Leucocyte separation and transfusion. *Br J Haematol* 28:271-275, 1974.

28. Schiffer CA: Principles of granulocyte transfusion therapy. *Med Clin N Am* 61:1119-1131, 1977.

29. Workman RD, Faville RJ, Strate RG, et al: Granulocyte transfusions for patients with severe thermal burns. *Transfusion* 18:142-148, 1978.

30. Vallejos C, McCredie KB, Bodey GP, et al: White blood cell transfusions for control of infections in neutropenic patients. *Transfusion* 15:28-32, 1975.

31. Graw RG, Herzig G, Perry S, et al: Normal granulocyte transfusion therapy. *N Engl J Med* 287:367-371, 1972.

32. Lalezari P: *The Granulocyte: Function and Clinical Utilization,* Greenwalt TJ, Jamieson GA (eds). New York, Alan R. Liss, Inc, 1977, p 209.

33. Drew SI, Carter BM, Terasaki PI, et al: Cell surface antigens detected on mature and leukemic granulocytic populations by cytotoxicity testing. *Tissue Antigens* 12:75-86, 1978.

34. Marsh, WL, Øyen R, Nichols ME: Kidd blood group antigens of leukocytes and platelets. *Transfusion* 14:378-381, 1974.

35. van de Wiel TWM, van de Wiel-Dorfmeyer H, van Loghem JJ: Studies on platelet antibodies in man. *Vox Sang* 6:641-688, 1961.

36. Aster RH, Cooper HE, Singer DL: Simplified complement fixation

test for the detection of platelet antibodies in human serum. *J. Lab Clin Med* 63:161-172, 1964.

37. Aster RH, Levin RH, Cooper H, et al: Complement-fixing platelet isoantibodies in serum of transfused persons. Correlation of antibodies with platelet survival in thrombocytopenic patients. *Transfusion* 4:428-440, 1964.

38. Dausset J, Colin M, Colombani J: Immune platelet isoantibodies. *Vox Sang* 5:4-31, 1960.

39. Mittal KK, Mickey MR, Singal DP, et al: Serotyping for homotransplantation XVIII. Refinement of microdroplet lymphocyte cytotoxicity test. *Transplantation* 6:913-928, 1968.

40. Amos DB: Freezing and thawing lymphocytes, in Ray JE, Hare DB, Pederson PD, et al (eds): *NIAID Manual of Tissue Typing Techniques.* DHEW Publication No (NIH) 76-545, 1976, p 186.

41. Shaw JF: Preliminary screening and tentative identification of HLA lymphocytotoxic antibodies in a hospital blood bank, in Ray RG, Hare DB, Pederson PD, et al (eds): *NIAID Manual of Tissue Typing Techniques.* DHEW Publication No. (NIH) 76-545, 1976. p 161.

42. van dem Borne AEG, Verheugt WA, Oosterhof F, et al: A simple immunofluorescence test for the detection of platelet antibodies. *Br J Haematol* 39:195-207, 1978.

43. Brand A. van Leeuwen A, Eernisse JG, et al: Platelet transfusion therapy. Optimal donor selection with a combination of lymphocytotoxicity and platelet fluorescence tests. *Blood* 51:781-788, 1978.

44. Gockerman JP, Bowman RP, Conrad ME: Detection of platelet isoantibodies by ^{3}H-Serotonin platelet release and its clinical application to the problem of platelet matching. *J Clin Invest* 55:75-83, 1975.

45. Hirschman RJ, Shulman NR: The use of platelet serotonin release as a sensitive method for detecting anti-platelet antibodies and a plasma anti-platelet factor in patients with idiopathic thrombocytopenic purpura. *Br J Haematol* 24:793-802, 1973.

46. Horowitz HI, Rappaport HI, Young RC, et al: Change in platelet factor 3 as a means of demonstrating immune reactions involving platelets: its use as a test for quinidine induced thrombocytopenia. *Transfusion* 5:336-343, 1965.

47. Karpatkin S, Siskind GW: In vitro detection of platelet antibody in patients with idiopathic thrombocytopenic purpura and systemic lupus erythematosus. *Blood* 33:795-802, 1969.

48. Deykin D, Hellerstein LJ: The assessment of drug dependent and isoimmune antiplatelet antibodies by the use of platelet aggregometry. *J Clin Invest* 51:3142-3153, 1972.

49. Mueller-Eckhardt D, Schulz G, Dienst C, et al: ^{125}I-Anti-immunoglobulin test: A new tool for the detection of drug allergic platelet antibodies. *Vox Sang* 34:43-45, 1978.

50. Yankee RA, Grumet FC, Rogensine GN: Platelet transfusion therapy: The selection of compatible platelet donors for refractory patients by lymphocyte HLA typing. *N Engl J Med* 281:1208-1212, 1969.

51. Yankee RA, Graff KS, Dowing R: Selection of unrelated compatible platelet donors by lymphocyte HLA matching. *N Engl J Med* 288:760-764, 1973.

52. Lohrmann HP, Bull MI, Decter JA, et al: Platelet transfusions from HLA compatible unrelated donors to alloimmunized patients. *Ann Int Med* 80:9-14, 1974.

53. Thorsby E, Helgesen A, Gjemdal T: Repeated platelet transfusion from HLA compatible unrelated and sibling donors. *Tissue Antigens* 2:397-404, 1972.

54. Mittal KK, Ruder EA, Green D: Matching of histocompatibility (HLA) antigens for platelet transfusion. *Blood* 47:31-41, 1976.

55. Gmür J, von Felte A, Frick P: Platelet support in polysensitized patients: Role of HLA specificities and crossmatch testing for donor selection. *Blood* 51:903-909, 1978.

56. Duquesnoy RJ, Testin J, Aster H: Variable expression of w4 and w6 on platelets: Possible relevance to platelet transfusion therapy of alloimmunized thrombocytopenic patients. *Trans Proc* 9:1829-1831, 1977.

57. Aster RH, Szatkowski N, Liebert M, et al: Expression of HLA B12, HLA B8, w4, and w6 on platelets. *Trans Proc* 9:1695-1696, 1977.

58. Aster RH, Jandl JH: Platelet sequestration in man. II. Immunological and clinical studies. *J Clin Invest* 43:856-868, 1964.

59. Minev M: Differences in the immunogenicity of the HLA antigens. *Vox Sang* 29:433-439, 1975.

60. Opelz G, Mickey MR, Teraski PI: Blood transfusions and unresponsiveness to HLA. *Transplantation* 16:649-654, 1973.

61. Bucher U, de Weck A, Spengler H, et al: Platelet transfusions: Shortened survival of HLA identical platelets and failure of in vitro detection of anti-platelet antibodies after multiple transfusions. *Vox Sang* 25:187-192, 1973.

62. Herzig RH, Herzig GP, Bull MI, et al: Correction of poor platelet transfusion responses with leukocyte-poor HLA-matched platelet concentrates. *Blood* 46:743-750, 1975.

63. Wu KK, Hoak JC, Koepke JA, et al: Selection of compatible platelet donors: A prospective evaluation of three crossmatching techniques. *Transfusion* 17:638-642, 1977.

64. Duquesnoy RJ, Filip DJ, Tomasulo PA, et al: Role of HLA-C matching in histocompatible platelet transfusion therapy of alloimmunized thrombocytopenic patients. *Trans Proc* 9:1827-1828, 1977.

65. Svejgaard, A: Isoantigenic systems of human blood platelets. *Ser Haematol* 3:5-87, 1969.

66. Shulman NR, Marder VJ, Hiller MC, et al: Platelet and leukocyte isoantigens and their antibodies: serologic, physiologic and clinical studies. *Prog Haemat* 4:222-304, 1964.

67. Shulman NR, Aster RH, Leitner A, et al: Immunoreactions involving platelets. V. Post transfusion purpura due to a complement fixing antibody against a genetically controlled platelet antigen. A proposed mechanism for thrombocytopenia and its relevance in 'autoimmunity.' *J Clin Invest* 40:1597-1612, 1961.

68. Slichter SJ, Harker LA: Transfused platelet compatibility: Selection by HLA vs crossmatching technique. *Blood* 46:163, 1975 (abstract).

69. Filip DJ, Duquesnoy RJ, Aster RH: Predictive value of crossmatching for transfusion of platelet concentrates to alloimmunized recipients. *Am J Hematol* 1:471-479, 1976.

70. Herzig RH, Terasaki PI, Trapani GP, et al: The relationship between donor recipient lymphocytotoxicity and the transfusion response using HLA matched platelet concentrates. *Transfusion* 17:657-661, 1977.

71. Wu KK, Hoak JC, Thompson JS, et al: Use of platelet aggregometry in selection of compatible platelet donors. *N Engl J Med* 292:130-133, 1975.

72. Roy AJ, Jaffe N, Djerassi I: Prophylactic platelet transfusions in children with acute leukemia: a dose response study. *Transfusion* 13:283-290, 1973.

73. Gaydos LA, Freireich EJ, Mantel J: The quantitative relation between platelet count and hemorrhage in patients with acute leukemia. *Transfusion* 266:905-909, 1962.

74. Higby DJ, Cohen E, Hollan JF, et al: The prophylactic treatment of thrombocytopenic leukemic patients with platelets: a double blind study. *Transfusion* 14:440-446, 1974.

75. Patel IP, Ambinder E, Holland JF, et al: In vitro and in vivo comparison of single donor platelets and multiple-donor pooled platelet transfusions in leukemic patients. *Transfusion* 18:116-118, 1978.

76. Milgrom F, Palester M, Wozniczko G, et al: Complement fixing leucocyte antibodies. *Vox Sang* 2:263-269, 1957.

77. Logue GL, Kurlander R, Pepe P, et al: Antibody dependent lymphocyte mediated granulocyte cytotoxicity in man. *Blood* 51:97-107, 1978.

78. Hasegawa T, Graw RG, Terasaki PI: A microgranulocyte cytotoxicity test. *Transplantation* 15:492-498, 1973.

79. Caplan SN, Berkman EM, Babior BM: Cytotoxins against a granulocyte antigen system: detection by a new method employing cytochalasin B treated cells. *Vox Sang* 33:206-211, 1977.

80. Clay ME, McCullough J: Studies of the granulocyte cytotoxicity assay, abstracted. *Transfusion* 18:395, 1978.

81. Verheugt FWA, von dem Borne AEG, van Noord-Bokhorst JC, et al: Serological, immunochemical and immunocytological properties of granulocyte antibodies. *Vox Sang* 35:294-303, 1978.

82. Verheught FWA, von dem Borne AEG, Decary F, et al: The detection of granulocyte alloantibodies with an indirect immunofluorescence test. *Br J Haematol* 36:533-544, 1977.

83. Lalezari, P, Radel E: Neutrophil specific antigens: Immunology and clinical significance. *Sem Hematol* 11:281-290, 1974.

84. Jiang A, Lalezari P: A microtechnique for detection of leukocyte agglutinins. *J Immunol Meth* 7:103-108, 1975.

85. Zmiejewski CM: EDTA agglutination assay, in Ray JG, Hare DG, Pederson, PD, et al (eds): *NIAID Manual of Tissue Typing Techniques.* DHEW Publication No. (NIH) 76-545, 1976, p 18.

86. Thompson JS, Severson CD, Coppleson LW, et al: Leukocyte capillary agglutination, in Teraski PI: *Histocompatibility Testing.* Copenhagen, Munksgaard, 1970, p 587.

87. Boxer AB, Stossel TP: Effects of anti-human neutrophil antibodies in vitro. *J Clin Invest* 53:1534-1543, 1974.

88. Laleli YR, Bilezikian SB, Tsan MF, et al: Immunological reactions involving leukocytes: I. detection of antibodies to human granulocytes by measurement of the metabolic events associated with phagocytosis. *J Hopkins Med J* 138:43-47, 1976.

89. Eyre HJ, Goldstein IM, Perry S, et al: Leukocyte transfusions: function of transfused granulocytes from donors with chronic myelocytic leukemia. *Blood* 36:432-442, 1970.

90. Goldstein IM, Eyre HJ, Terasaki PI, et al: Leukocyte transfusions: Role of leukocyte alloantibodies in determining transfusion response. *Transfusion* 11:19-24, 1971.

91. Appelbaum FR, Trapani RJ, Graw RG: Consequences of prior alloimmunization during granulocyte transfusion. *Transfusion* 17: 460-464, 1976.

92. Ungerleider RS, Appelbaum FR, Trapani RJ, et al: Lack of predictive value of antileukocyte antibody screening in granulocyte transfusion therapy. *Transfusion* 19:90-94, 1979.

93. Graw RG, Goldstein IM, Eyre HJ, et al: Histocompatibility testing for leucocyte transfusion. *Lancet* 2:77-78, 1970.

94. Koza I, Holland JF, Cohen E: Histocompatible leukocyte transfusion during granulocytopenia. *Neoplasma* 18:185-191, 1971.

95. Ozturk GE, Terasaki PI: Non HLA lymphocytotoxic antibodies in disease, abstracted. Fourth Annual Meeting of the Am Assoc Clin Histocompat Testing, 1978, p 69.

96. Pruzanski W, Armstrong M, Urowitz MB: Heterogeneity of cold and warm reacting cytotoxins against lymphocytes, granulocytes and monocytes in rheumatic diseases. *Clin Immun and Immunopath* 11:142-146, 1978.

97. Hasegawa T, Bergh OJ, Terasaki PI, et al: Occurrence of granulocyte cytotoxins and agglutinins. *Transfusion* 15:226-230, 1975.

98. Schiffer CA, Bucholz DH, Aisner J, et al: Clinical experience with transfusion of granulocytes obtained by continuous flow filtration leukopheresis. *Am J Med* 58:373-381, 1975.

99. Ward HN: Pulmonary infiltrates associated with leukoagglutinin transfusion reactions. *Ann Int Med* 73:689-694, 1970.

100. Schiffer CA, Aisner J, Wiernik PH: Frozen autologous platelet transfusion for patients with leukemia. *N Engl J Med* 299:7-13, 1977.